Spanish Flu

I0370039

The Deadliest Pandemic That the Human Race Has Faced

(The History and Legacy of the World's Deadliest Influenza Outbreak)

Andrew Lawrence

Published By **Phil Dawson**

Andrew Lawrence

All Rights Reserved

Spanish Flu: The Deadliest Pandemic That the Human Race Has Faced (The History and Legacy of the World's Deadliest Influenza Outbreak)

ISBN 978-1-7753142-6-4

No part of this guidebook shall be reproduced in any form without permission in writing from the publisher except in the case of brief quotations embodied in critical articles or reviews.

Legal & Disclaimer

The information contained in this book is not designed to replace or take the place of any form of medicine or professional medical advice. The information in this book has been provided for educational & entertainment purposes only.

The information contained in this book has been compiled from sources deemed reliable, and it is accurate to the best of the Author's knowledge; however, the Author cannot guarantee its accuracy and validity and cannot be held liable for any errors or omissions. Changes are periodically made to this book. You must consult your doctor or get professional medical advice before using any of the suggested remedies, techniques, or information in this book.

Upon using the information contained in this book, you agree to hold harmless the Author from and against any damages, costs, and expenses, including any legal fees potentially resulting from the application of any of the information provided by this guide. This disclaimer applies to any damages or injury caused by the use and application, whether directly or indirectly, of any advice or information presented, whether for breach of contract, tort, negligence, personal injury, criminal intent, or under any other cause of action.

You agree to accept all risks of using the information presented inside this book. You need to consult a professional medical practitioner in order to ensure you are both able and healthy enough to participate in this program.

Table Of Contents

Chapter 1: Origin Of The Influenza Pandemic Of 1918-19

The sudden outbreak of the virus in 1918-19 became referred to as flu Pandemic. It modified into one of the most extreme influenza outbreaks of the 20th century. In terms of absolute numbers of deaths, it have become one of the maximum devastating pandemics in human facts. Influenza is due to a pandemic it actually is transmitted from character to individual. An outbreak can rise up from which the populace has no immunity if a brand new stress of flu virus emerges. The flu pandemic of 1918-19 affected populations to a large proportion. An influenza virus, known as flu type A subtype H1N1, is currently confirmed to have turn out to be the beginning location of the intense mortality of the outbreak, which introduced on an expected 25 million deaths, despite the reality that some researchers have expected it brought about as many as forty-50 million deaths. The pandemic befell in 3 waves. The first reputedly originated in ancient March 1918, sooner or later of World War I. Though it stays doubtful at which the virus first surfaced, it unexpectedly spread through Western Europe, and with the useful resource of using July it had spread to Poland. The preliminary wave of flu modified into moderate. However, a shape of sickness were diagnosed to be because of it, and this type regarded in August 1918. Pneumonia advanced after the initial signs of this influenza. As an example, at Camp Devens, Massachusetts, U.S., six days after the number one case of flu became cited, that there were 6,674 times. The subsequent wave of the pandemic occurred in the subsequent wintry climate, and from the spring that the virus had run its software. In every waves form of half of of of the deaths had been amongst 20-forty-yr-olds, an unusual mortality era pattern for flu. Outbreaks of this influenza occurred in almost each inhabited part of the arena, first in vents, then dispersing from town to metropolis for the duration of the primary transport routes. India is concept to have endured at 12.Five million deaths inside the path of the pandemic, and moreover the illness attained far flung islands within the South Pacific, collectively with New Zealand and Samoa. Roughly 550,000 people died. Most deaths happened within the path of the 1/3 and 2nd waves. Outbreaks of flu came about with virulence within the Twenties.

Epidemic

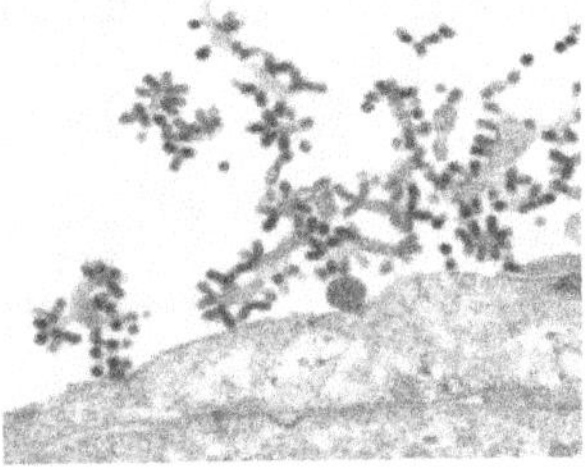

The epidemic is an incident of disorder it truely is speedy excessive. If the superiority of a pandemic takes place over a huge geographical area (e.G., globally), it's miles known as an endemic. The upward thrust and fall within the outbreak occurrence of infectious illness are probably to be took place through using the shipping of an effective dose of the infectious agent from an inflamed man or woman to a willing character. Following a virulent disease has escalated, the affected server populace includes a small sufficient percentage of susceptible people that reintroduction of this sickness may not reason a trendy outbreak. Considering that the parasite populace can't replicate itself on this form of bunch population, the host populace as an entire is evidence in opposition to the epidemic sickness, a phenomenon termed herd resistance. After an endemic, the host populace will revert into a state of susceptibility because of (1) the corrosion of human resistance; (2) the removal of resistant human beings bypassing, and (three) the influx of prone human beings via the usage of transport. With the years the people as a whole become greater willing. The time elapsing among outbreak peaks differs from some other and is changeable. From the overdue twentieth century that the definition of the outbreak emerge as extended to embody outbreaks of any continual disorder or infection (e.G., cardiovascular sickness or weight troubles). The expression outbreak may be earmarked for illness among humans; an epidemic of contamination among animals other than guy is referred to as as epizootic.

Influenza

This is likewise known as a serious viral, grippe, or flu. This ailment of the top or decrease respiration tract is indicated with the beneficial aid of fever, chills, and a generalized feeling of ache and prone factor within the muscles, similarly to various tiers of ache on the pinnacle and gut.

A Sequence Of Influenza Infection

This is any of the numerous assets of influenza viruses from the family Orthomyxoviridae (a collection of RNA viruses). Flu viruses were classified as kinds A, B, C, D. These massive types typically produce comparable signs however are unrelated antigenically, in fact so infection with one kind confers no resistance in opposition to the others. The A viruses cause the amazing flu epidemics, together with the B germs cause smaller localized outbreaks. C viruses motive a moderate sickness. Influenza D viruses are not diagnosed to contaminate human beings and had been discovered simplest in cows. Influenza viruses are categorised into subtypes, and subtypes of influenza A and the 2 influenza B are cut up into breeds. Subtypes of influenza A are remarkable specially at the idea of ground antigens (overseas proteins) --hemagglutinin (H) and neuraminidase (N). Cases of flu subtypes include H1N1, H5N1, and H3N2. Strains of influenza strains and B of flu subtypes are further prominent with the aid of the use of versions inside the molecular association.

Evolution And Virulence Of Influenza Infection

Between outbreaks, the pandemics viruses undergo continuously, speedy improvement (a gadget referred to as antigenic glide), which may be powered with the useful useful resource of mutations within the genes encoding antigen proteins. Gradually, the viruses experience big evolutionary change by way of using manner of obtaining a trendy genome phase from a special flu virus (antigenic shift), effectively becoming a cutting-edge subtype. Animals facilitate evolution. If a pig is concurrently inflamed with extremely good influenza viruses, like human, swine, and avian traces, genetic reassortment may want to seem. This technique contributes to new lines of influenza A. Recently surfaced flu viruses are willing to be first of all exceptionally infectious and infectious in human beings because of the truth that they have novel antigens to the body does now not have any prepared immune safety (i.E., present antibodies). After an crucial percentage of people develop resistance through the introduction of antibodies able to preventing the emblem-new virus, the infectiousness and virulence of this virus lower. Although outbreaks of flu viruses are normally maximum lethal to immature children and the aged, the casualty price in humans among a while 20 and forty is from time to time immoderate, no matter the fact that the sufferers get remedy. This phenomenon is idea to be attributed to the hyper-response of their immune machine to new traces of the flu virus. Response results inside the overproduction of inflammatory chemical substances known as cytokines. The discharge of immoderate portions of those molecules induces contamination that is acute. People whose immune structures are not definitely superior (like toddlers) or are faded (similar to the older) can't create this form of deadly immune response.

Pandemics And Epidemics

Influenza pandemics are predicted to upward push up on a mean of every 50 a few years. Epidemics can also seem and the flu seems yearly occasionally. A pandemic can take location interior a depend variety of weeks, as speedy as influenza a virulent disease undergoes an antigenic exchange. The flu pandemic of 1918-19, the very unfavourable flu outbreak in facts and the various most acute illness pandemics that ever struck, become due to a subtype of influenza known as H1N1. In this occasion, an expected 25 million human beings international-enormous died of this so-called Spanish influenza, which changed into notably suggested in Spain however originated from Kansas, U.S.

Pandemics of flu were immoderate. For instance, influenza A subtype H2N2, or the 1957 influenza pandemic, reputedly started in East Asia early in 1957, and through midyear it had became round the world. The outbreak persevered to a virus amount until roughly the middle of 1958 and brought on an predicted 1 million to two million deaths globally. Following 10 some years of development that generated every 12 months epidemics, the 1957 flu vanished in 1968, clearly to get replaced with a ultra-modern influenza A subtype, H3N2. This virus is in flow. The influenza outbreak of 1968 has been the zero.33-biggest flu pandemic of the 20 th century additionally delivered about an anticipated 1 million to four million deaths. In 1997 a form of avian flu, or fowl flu, virus woke up among domesticated fowl in Hong Kong, then infected some humans, killing some of them. The real identical virus, H5N1, reappeared in one of the poultry flocks in Southeast Asia through the wintry weather of 2003-04, infecting some humans fatally. It hasoccasionally reappeared, notably talking in wild birds, domestic fowl, and people. A lot of subtypes of hen influenza viruses had been appeared, which include H7N2, H7N3, and H9N2.

An epidemic of a stress of H1N1 occurred in 2009. Initially called swine flu because the virus has been presupposed to were transmitted to humans from pigs; the disorder to start with broke out in Mexico and in the long run dispersed to the us. The H1N1 virus that introduced at the epidemic became discovered to private genetic cloth from human, avian, and 2 extraordinary swine flu viruses. The 2009 H1N1 epidemic end up not as deadly due to the fact the pandemic of 1918-19. The virus has been unfold and instead infectious. The pandemic possibility of this new H1N1 virus has been made apparent to the worldwide community from the World Health Organization (WHO), which broadcasted degree 5 pandemic signs on April 29, 2009. This triggered the implementation of discount strategies in international locations, to treatment facilities. Despite a number of these steps, the virus persevered to unfold. On June eleven, 2009, after an boom in times in Chile, Australia, and the UK, WHO extended the H1N1 alert diploma from five to 6, which means that that that the outbreak modified into formally added a virulent disease. From 2010 people in over 209 worldwide places had been affected. It modified into the first influenza pandemic of the twenty first century. In the us, the extended ranges of illness placed thru the 2009 pandemic had been not detected once more till 2018. Studies have encouraged that all the 4 historic flu pandemics changed into preceded with the aid of way of a La Niña event:a shift in global climate conditions associated with cool sea ground temperatures from the Pacific Ocean that some scientists speculate should have shifted the migratory kinds of birds, probably developing their interactions with home animals and empowering hereditary range and the increase of latest pandemic traces of flu viruses.

Influenza Pandemic Preparedness

Because flu epidemics and pandemics can devastate areas of the planet short, WHO monitors flu sickness pastime on a international scale. This remark is useful for collecting facts that may be employed to prepare vaccines and that can be disseminated to fitness centers in states wherein seasonal flu outbreaks will in all likelihood rise up. Tracking thru WHO pandemics performs a large element in stopping and making geared up for epidemics. In case a flu virus appears, WHO adheres to its pandemic preparedness software. This approach incorporates six degrees of pandemic alert. Phases 1-3, which might be the levels in preparedness, are all made to prevent or encompass outbreaks which have been modest. In these early ranges, remoted incidences of each animal-to-human transmissions of a flu virus were detected and supply caution indicators that an epidemic has pandemic capability. Little outbreaks of the disease may also moreover arise resulting, from times of transmission. Stage 3 signs and symptoms to states which are stricken by the execution of attempts are required to protect in opposition to an epidemic. Phases five and four have been characterised in mitigating the outbreak via urgency. Confirmed human-to-human viral transmission, collectively with the persistent contamination in human groups that unfold in order that ailment transmission among individuals occurred in best two states, shows that a pandemic is drawing close. Stage 6 is characterized with the aid of the use of contamination and transmission of the virus amongst people. Influenza pandemics take region in waves. Consequently, while infection hobby decreases a degree, it is probably discovered by some other segment of a immoderate occurrence of illness. Because of this, flu pandemics might also additionally persist for a length of weeks.

Transmission And Migraines

People of each age can also additionally get affected; but, the superiority of this illness is one of the adults and youngsters. Illness is transmitted from character to man or woman on this manner as inhalation of droplets principal to coughing and coughing. Since the virus debris gain access, they destroy and attack the epithelial cells, which line the respiration tract, bronchial tubes, and trachea. The incubation duration of the infection is one or days, and the symptoms are unexpected, with abrupt and unique misery, fatigue, and muscular aches. The temperature rises rapid to 38-forty °C (one 0 one-104 °F). Acute aches for the duration of the body and a headache are determined by using using a sense of rawness in the throat or aggravation. A few times the fever begins offevolved to drop, and the individual starts offevolved offevolved offevolved to get better. Feelings of fatigue can be amazing and accompany symptoms like coughing and nasal discharge. Complications like pneumonia or pneumonia may additionally get up among humans and might purpose loss of life.

Treatment And Prevention

The antiviral medicinal capsules rimantadine and amantadine have outcomes on instances of influenza amongst this type A virus. But immunity to those marketers has already been detected, thereby reducing their efficacy. A extra extremely-current class of medication, the neuraminidase inhibitors, which embody oseltamivir (Tamiflu) and zanamivir (Relenza), changed into launched in the late Nineties; the ones tablets inhibit every the influenza A and B viruses. Aside from this, an consumption of fluids, bed rest, and using analgesics is recommended. It's advised as remedy of illnesses with aspirin is associated with Reye syndrome, that kids and young adults with the flu not to take shipping of aspirin. Injection of a vaccine can also bolster protection in opposition to the flu. These germs are produced in chick embryos; arrangements that have been normal incorporate some of the ones a subtypes and the kind B flu virus. Security from 1 vaccination lasts yearly, and vaccination may be endorsed for those people which might be vulnerable to flu or whose scenario can also need to purpose headaches. But immunization in wholesome humans is advised. Advances within the comprehension of influenza and flu generation enabled the increase of a ordinary flu vaccine effective at defensive people in the direction of masses of flu subtypes.

To be capable of save you chook influenza viruses which might be human-infecting out of mutating into more risky subtypes, public health authorities attempt to restriction the viral "reservoir" in which antigenic alternate can also rise up by means of way of ordering the destruction of infected chicken flocks.

Pandemic

Pandemic is attached to the geographical place and it'd become affecting a superb percentage of the planet's population over the direction of many months. Pandemics originate from epidemics, that may be outbreaks of sickness restricted to a unmarried component, like a country. To make certain that a post-duration is probably found through another segment of excessive sickness occurrence, mainly the ones concerning flu, pandemics take location in waves. Diseases like flu can spread in a depend of days. Numerous factors facilitate the unfold of illness, which include an improved quantity of human-to-human transmission of this infection infectiousness of this consultant, and way of shipping. Diseases that rise up in animals motive the great majority. Therefore, at the same time as a modern infectious agent or sickness happens in creatures, surveillance agencies placed inner impacted areas are answerable for alerting the World Health Organization (WHO) and moreover for cautiously monitoring the conduct of this infectious agent and additionally the motion and unfold of this infection. WHO video display devices illness movement on a international scale with the aid of manner of a network of surveillance facilities determined in international locations. In the case of flu, WHO has organized a virulent disease preparedness plan that includes six degrees of pandemic alert, summarized as follows:

•Stage 1: the smallest degree of pandemic alert; suggests an influenza virus, likely genuinely regarded or previously gift, is circulating amongst creatures. The danger of transmission to human beings is decreased.

•Stage 2: remoted incidences of animal-to-human transmission of this virus have been detected, suggesting that the virus has pandemic ability.

•Stage three: characterised through manner of little outbreaks of disease, usually because of numerous instances of animal-to-human transmission, notwithstanding the truth that restrained capability for human-to-human transmission may be gift.

•Stage 4: supported human-to-human viral transmission which ends up in sustained ailment in human companies. At this issue, containment of the virus is deemed hopeless however there's an inevitable pandemic. The implementation of manage strategies to save you extra unfold is highlighted in regions of the planet.

•Stage five: indicated with human-to-human illness transmission in first-class states, signaling that a virulent disease is drawing near and that deliver of stockpiled pills and implementation of techniques to manipulate the illness desires to be completed with urgency.

•Stage 6: characterised via sustained and large disorder transmission among people.

When WHO updates a virus alert from stage four to diploma five, it functions as a signal to global locations to execute the strategies which are appropriate. Pandemics of illnesses like cholera, plague, and flu have done a element in forming human cultures. Examples of essential historic pandemics comprise the plague outbreak of the Portuguese Empire within the 6th century CE; the Black Death, that originated in China and unfold all through Europe from the 14th century; at the aspect of the flu pandemic of 1918-19, that originated from the U.S. Kingdom of Kansas and unfold into Europe, Asia, and islands in the South Pacific. Now several illnesses take area on a global scale persist in a excessive degree of incidence, even though pandemics are characterised by way of the use of their incidence on a period of time, and maybe transmitted among individuals. Such illnesses represented in modern-day pandemics consist of AIDS, due to HIV (human immunodeficiency virus), which may be transmitted directly amongst humans; and malaria, because of parasites in the genus Plasmodium, which can be transferred from one creature to each specific thru mosquitoes, which feed at the blood of inflamed individuals.

Influenza pandemics are expected to get up about each 50 a long time, no matter the fact that the duration in its prevalence has been shorter than that. After 191–nine, you could find actually extra flu pandemics: the 1957 Asian flu and the 1968 Hong Kong influenza pandemic. Until approximately 1958, an epidemic arose that grow to be liable for over one million deaths. The influenza pandemic occurred in 2009 while a subtype of virus unfold at some stage in areas of the earth. Between March 2009 and mid-January 2010, H1N1 deaths have been recommended. In March 2020 an epidemic of a Novel coronavirus known as immoderate acute breathing syndrome coronavirus-2 (SARS-CoV2) have become added with the aid of WHO officers. Infection with SARS-CoV2 generated an contamination referred to as coronavirus disorder 2019 (COVID-19); the illness modified into characterized through the use of cough, fever, and shortness of breath. The outbreak started out at Wuhan, China in 2019, as speedy as a affected person with disabilities modified into admitted to a medical institution. In the subsequent few weeks, the sort of human beings climbed in ratio, at the side of the spread of the Wuhan Disease into different regions of China. By 2020, COVID-19 had protected america and Europe thru vacationers. From the time the epidemic have become brought, instances of COVID-19 were located worldwide. There have been showed cases and approximately five,000 deaths.

Chapter 2: The Origin And History Of Spanish Flu

This flu's supply has been debated. The Claude Hannoun Pasteur Institute has posited that the virus originated in China, dispersed through troop movements, and from there, to Boston and Kansas, then to Brest, France. Here's a timeline of the Spanish Flu rallied round the world.

April 1917 - the U.S. Enters World War I with 378,000 men in the navy, this could rapid swell to limitless guys.

June 1917 - to elevate the amount of men, there may be a draft created. The army creates each home 25,000 to fifty five,000 guys, 32 schooling facilities.

March 1918 - That wide variety extended 5-fold constant with week later. Sporadic instances of the influenza start acting some one of a kind region inside the U.S., additionally in Europe and Asia.

April 1918 - that the point out of this influenza appears describing three deaths and 18 times.

May 1918 - that the U.S. Commenced shipping hundreds upon lots of troops to Europe. Due to the conflict, censors at Germany, England, France, and the U.S. Have been blocking information of this epidemic, leaving impartial Spain to file the disease. This is the way it were given the name, the "Spanish Flu." The virus spreads from Europe into North America, Asia, Africa, Brazil, islands within the South Pacific, in addition to indigenous tribes residing within the Arctic Circle.

September 1918 - every other wave of this virus emerges, which has a higher fatality rate than the previous wave. It developed in an Army facility, also in a Navy facility in Boston virtually outdoor the town.

This tide is liable for the majority of the deaths inside the virus, with 12,000 people loss of life from the U.S. Through September. The New York City Board of Health required that instances of influenza be stated and patients are remoted, every in home or in a health facility. To get a Liberty Bonds parade, hundred,000 people acquire lower back in Philadelphia, and day's 635 instances of the flu are said. Theaters, church homes, and the metropolis dictate faculties have been closed.

October 1918 - 195,000 Americans die of the flu in this month. There's a scarcity of nurses because of the reality that maximum are presently serving. The American Red Cross Chicago Chapter troubles a call for volunteers to nurse the sick. Colleges and film theaters near, and public gatherings are prohibited via the use of them. Legislation in Chicago drops with the aid of using 40 three percent. Is made to region away corpses and additionally a secondhand vehicle maker calls for packing crates to be carried out as coffins. San Francisco urges that face mask are worn through of its citizens out in people, and in NYC, shipbuilding is down with the resource of forty percent because of absenteeism.

November 1918 - Soldiers are added instances of the influenza, and reduce lower returned home through the perception of the war. Signals are located thru officials at Salt Lake City. In France, the armistice is signed on November 11, 1918, finishing WWI. U.S. President Woodrow Wilson collapses after coming down with the flu.

January 1919 - a wave of the virus emerges, killing masses people. Between January 1st and the 5th, 1,800 influenza instances which might be new are skilled via the usage of San Francisco, and one zero one human beings perish. New York City reviews 706 times and sixty seven deaths.

August 1919 - the Influenza pandemic comes to a surrender due to the fact human beings who have been inflamed perished or advanced resistance.

March 1997 - onMarch twenty first, 1997, a bit of writing is posted in Science Magazine. Researchers at the Armed Forces Institute of Pathology tested lung tissue acquired via way of a soldier that died in 1918 of this influenza. They cease that even though the influenza virus is super, that, "The hemagglutinin receptor suits closest to swine flu viruses, demonstrating that this virus came to humans through pigs."

February 2004 - Researchers on the Scripps Institute in La Jolla, California and in England's Medical Research Council finish that the 1918 virus may also want to have jumped without delay from birds to people, bypassing dinosaurs completely. This also can give an explanation for the virulence of this disease.

October 2005 - Scientists in the Armed Forces Institute of Pathology order the entire genome of this virus through the use of studying cells taken inside the whole frame of a flu sufferer whose frame become preserved in permafrost due to the reality he have been buried in 1918.

Etymology

Despite its call, epidemiological and ancient information can't turn out to be privy to the foundation of the flu. The source of this "Spanish influenza" understand comes out of the pandemic's spread to Spain from France in November 1918. Spain wasn't concerned having stayed unbiased, and hadn't enforced censorship all through wartime. Newspapers had been free to record the epidemic's effects, just like the grave contamination of King Alfonso XIII, and such extensively-spread memories generated a faux perception. Almost a century after the influenza struck in 1918--1920, the World Health Oganization (WHO) known as on scientists, countrywide governments and the clicking to study tremendous practices in discovering smooth human infectious illnesses to reduce pointless adverse effects on states, economies and people. More present day phrases with this virus embody the "1918 flu pandemic," the"1918 influenza pandemic," or versions of them.

Hypotheses Concerning The Origin

British Troops In France

The UK troop health facility and staging camp at Étaples in Virologist John Oxford has speculated France as being inside the center of the flu. His evaluation decided that with high mortality, which brought on signs and symptoms like the flu, the Étaples camp have been struck with the beneficial aid of the begin of a ailment at 1916. Based on Oxford, a comparable outbreak occurred in March 1917 at navy barracks at Alders, and army pathologists afterwards placed out those untimely outbreaks had been the correct identical illness because the 1918 influenza. Hospital and the camp have been best net websites for dispersing the virus. The health facility dealt with 100,000 infantrymen, patients of conflict, and chemical assaults. It become domestic to a piggery, and fowl had been added in for meals resources in villages. His organization and oxford declared that a metric virus, sailed to pigs and harbored in critters, mutated. A report posted in 2016 at the Journal of the Chinese Medical Association decided signs that the 1918 virus changed into circulating inside the European armies for months and probable years prior to the 1918 pandemic.

United States

There have been bulletins that the outbreak originated in the United States. Historian Alfred W. Crosby said in 2003 that the influenza originated in Kansas, and famous author John M. Barry described a January 1918 outbreak in Haskell County, Kansas because the factor of beginning from his

2004 article. A 2018 analysis of tissue slides and clinical reports directed with the aid of evolutionary studies scientist Michael Worobec positioned proof opposite to the sickness bobbing up out of Kansas, as the ones instances had fewer deaths while in assessment with the scenario in NYC at exactly the precise same time body. The have a look at didn't discover signs and symptoms; even though it wasn't conclusive, the virus had a supply. Additionally, the haemagglutinin glycoproteins of the virus suggest that it had been spherical long until 1918 collectively with every other studies propose that the reassortment of the H1N1 virus likely took place in kind of 1915.

China

Among the areas of the world apparently encouraged from the 1918 influenza pandemic modified into China, wherein there might have been a quite moderate flu season in 1918 (despite the fact that that is disputed because of absence of data at some level within the Warlord Period of China, go to Around the arena). Studies have said that there were deaths in evaluation to particular regions of earth. This has brought on hypothesis that the 1918 influenza pandemic originated in China. Rates of influenza mortality in China in 1918 and the flu season might be clarified through the populace acquired immunity to the influenza virus. In 1993, the professional for the Pasteur Institute about the 1918 flu, Claude Hannoun, claimed the virus turned into likely to have come from China. It then mutated inside the USA near Boston and from there unfold to Brest, France, Europe's battlefields, Europe, and the planet with Allied soldiers and sailors as the primary disseminators. In 2014, historian Mark Humphries contended the mobilization of all employees to feature inside the lower back of the French and British lines might have been the beginning of the pandemic. Humphries, of the Memorial University of

Newfoundland in St. John's, based his options on in recent times unearthed statistics. He found proof turned into diagnosed with the aid of health officials identical to the flu. A document published in 2016 on the Journal of the Chinese Medical Association placed no symptoms and signs that the 1918 virus had been imported to Europe thru Chinese and Southeast Asian soldiers and employees, butinstead placed symptoms and signs of its glide in Europe preceding to the pandemic. The 2016 have a look at indicated that the very low flu mortality price (an expected 1/a thousand) determined one of the Chinese and Southeast Asian employees in Europe intended the deadly 1918 flu pandemic could not have originated from the ones personnel. A 2018 assessment of tissue slides and scientific reviews directed with the resource of evolutionary research scientist Michael Worobey placed proof contrary to the disease being allotted by manner of the usage of Chinese employees, noting that personnel entered Europe thru one-of-a-kind avenues, which did no longer cause detectable spread, making them now not going to have been the proper hosts.

Additional

Hannoun taken into consideration certainly one of a type hypotheses of supply, like Spain, Kansas, and Brest, as potential, however no longer possibly. Political scientist Andrew Price-Smith published information within the records in Austria, 1917.

Spread

When an infected character sneezes or coughs, million virus debris can disperse to human beings nearby. Troop moves of World War I and close quarters hastened each transmissions, and probably the pandemic and mutation that have been augmented. The lethality of the virus may additionally have improved. Some speculate that the soldiers' immune systems have been weakened, in addition to through malnourishment. An detail interior the superiority of the flu grow to be raised journey. Modern shipping structures made it an lousy lot a good deal much less tough for sailors, soldiers, or maybe vacationers to unfold the contamination. The following become refusal and lies via the usage of authorities.

The ailment have become discovered in Haskell County, Kansas, in January 1918, prompting community medical doctor Loring Miner to frighten that the US Public Health Service's instructional diary. About 4 March 1918, enterprise put together dinner Albert Gitchell, from Haskell County, stated sick at Fort Riley, a US army facility that at the time were schooling American troops inside the direction of World War I, making him the first recorded sufferer of the influenza. In days, guys within the camp had stated unwell. About 11 Queens were conquered by way of manner of the virus.

Everyone end up suffering to take steps to counter it but their movements had been criticized. In August 1918, a extra virulent stress regarded simultaneously in Brest, France; at Freetown, Sierra Leone; and at the U.S., in September, inside the Boston Navy Yard and Camp Devens (later renamed Fort Devens), form of 30 kilometers west of Boston. Other U.S. Army web sites had been speedy affected, as have been infantrymen being hauled to Europe. By returning infantrymen, the influenza carried there.

Mortality

Around The World

The influenza effected approximately 1 / four of the planet's populace. Estimates as to how many inflamed humans died range drastically, but the influenza come to be now not seemed due to the fact the various deadliest pandemics. A quote from 1991 claims that the virus killed among 25 and 39 million human beings. A 2005 estimate located the demise toll in 50 million (a whole lot less than three percent of the global population), and possibly as huge as one hundred million (extra than 5 percentage). However, a reassessment at 2018 envisioned the overall to be about 17 million, despite the fact that this turn out to be contested. With a global populace of 1.Eight to at the least one.Nine billion, the ones estimates correspond between 1 and six% of the population. This influenza killed more humans than The Black Death, that lasted longer, murdered a percentage of the arena's smaller population. The infection killed in regions of the planet. A few 12-17 million humans died more or less 5 percentage of the population, in India. The loss of life toll in India's British-dominated districts modified into thirteen.88 million. Arnold (2019) costs as a minimum 12 million deceased. Estimates for its death toll in China have various, which suggests the absence of business enterprise of health facts. The first quote of this Chinese lack of existence toll has been created in 1991 by way of way of Patterson and Pyle, which anticipated China desired a demise toll of amongst five and nine million. But research due to defective approach criticized this 1991 assessment, and studies have released estimates of a mortality rate in China. As an instance, Iijima in 1998 estimates that the death toll in China to be among 1 and 1.28 million in line with records accessible Chinese port cities. Since, Wataru Iijima notes,' Pyle and Patterson inner their studies 'The 1918 Influenza Pandemic' tried to gauge the quantity of deaths as a whole from the flu in China. They contended amongst four.Zero and nine.Five million human beings died in China, but this popular come to be mounted most effective at the idea that the passing price there has been 1.Zero--2.25 percentage in 1918, whilst you preserve in thoughts that China modified right into a terrible nation very similar to Indonesia and India in which the mortality price become of the acquisition.

Their evaluation wasn't primarily based mostly on any statistical statistics. The lower estimates of the Chinese lack of lifestyles toll derive from the minimal mortality charges, which were determined in Chinese port cities (through way of instance, Hong Kong) and moreover on the idea that terrible communications avoided the influenza from getting into the internal of China. But some contemporary post and newspaper workplace evaluations, similarly to critiques from missionary physicians, imply the influenza didn't penetrate the Chinese inner and that flu emerge as lousy in certain locations inside the geographical location of China.

23 million human beings have been affected; with at least deaths had been said with the useful resource of 390,000. From the Dutch East Indies (now Indonesia), 1.Five million had been speculated to have expired amongst 30 million human beings. In Tahiti, thirteen percent of the humans

died in some unspecified time in the future of a month. In the identical manner, in simplest months, 22 percent of the population of 38,000 died at Samoa. In New Zealand, the flu killed an expected 6,four hundred Pakeha and a pair of,500 nearby Maori in fourteen days, together with Māori expiring at 8 instances the price of Pakeha.

In Iran, the Mortality changed into quite immoderate:

•According to a quote, 8 to 22 percent of the populace, or regarding 902,4 hundred and a couple of,431,000 expired.

In the U.S., type of 28 percentage of the Populace of 1 zero five million have emerge as infected, and 500,000 to 850,000 expired (0.Forty 8 to 0.Eighty one percentage of the population). Native American tribes were tough hit. There were deaths amongst Americans. Alaskan village groups and complete Inuit expired in Alaska. 50,000 expired. In Britain, as many as in France,

Alves Back in Brazil, over four hundred,000. In Ghana, as a minimum one hundred,000 individuals were killed by using the flu epidemic. Tafari Makonnen (the close to destiny Haile Selassie, Emperor of Ethiopia) have become amongst those earliest Ethiopians who contracted flu but lived. Many of the subjects did not; expenses for deaths from the capital metropolis include even better or even five,000 to ten,000. In British Somaliland, 1 right expected that 7 percent of the populace died. This dying toll brought about from an contamination fee of the seriousness of these signs and symptoms and symptoms and moreover round 50%, suspected to be added on through storms. Symptoms in 1918 were uncommon causing flu. 1 contributor wrote, "Among the most superb of those complications modified into hemorrhage from mucous membranes, particularly from the nostril, stomach, and intestine. Bleeding from the ears and petechial hemorrhages in pores and skin moreover took place". The excellent majority of deaths were a secondary ailment, from pneumonia. By inducing hemorrhages and edema in the 15, the virus murdered people.

Patterns Of Fatality

Adults were killed through the usage of the pandemic. Back in 1918–1919, ninety nine percent of pandemic flu deaths from the U.S. Passed off in people underneath sixty 5, and nearly half of of deaths were in teenagers 20 to 40 years old. The mortality rate amongst human beings below sixty five had dwindled six-fold however ninety percent of deaths occurred in humans. Because the flu is typically deadly to people, like toddlers underneath age 2 and the immune compromised, this is uncommon. Back in 1918, older adults could probably have skilled partial safety brought on via exposure to the 1889-1890 influenza pandemic, known as the "Russian flu." Based on historian John M. Barry, the most uncovered of– "the ones probably, of the very in all likelihood", to perish -- were pregnant ladies. He cautioned in 13 researches of ladies inside the pandemic, the lack of existence fee ranged from 23 to 71 percentage. Of those pregnant girls who lived childbirth, over one-area (26 percentage) dropped the child. The unique oddity have become that the epidemic come to be regular on the summer time and fall (from the Northern Hemisphere); flu is usually worse within the wintry climate. Contemporary research has demonstrated that the virus to be particularly lethal because it turns on a cytokine typhoon (overreaction of the frame's immune device), which ravages the greater powerful immune device of young adults. The virus became retrieved with the aid of using the usage of 1 set of investigators within the our our bodies of creatures that had been transfected and sufferers with it. The creatures suffered innovative respiration failure and passing. Whereas the poorer reactions of adults and children caused deaths, the immune reactions of adults had been postulated to have shattered the whole frame. By consolidation, mortality has been specifically in situations. Cases comprised neural involvement that led every now and then to intellectual issues, and bacterial infections. Some deaths had been the end quit end result of malnourishment. A studies accomplished hired a mechanistic modeling method to test the three waves of the 1918 flu pandemic. They analyzed the factors that underlie variability of their importance and styles to styles of morbidity and mortality. Their evaluation shows that the purpose is supplied via versions in transmission pace, and moreover the model is internal plausible values. Another assessment via way of The et al. (2013) hired a clean epidemic version comprising three variables to infer the motive for the three waves of the 1918 flu pandemic. These variables have been closure and university beginning, temperature changes at some point of the outbreak, and individual adjustments in response to this outbreak. The results were examined by means of manner of using behavioral reactions, regardless of the reality that their modeling outcomes hooked up that each one three variables are substantial. A 2020 analysis observed that US towns, which performed huge and early non-clinical measures (quarantine and plenty of others.) continued no similarly detrimental economic outcomes due to imposing the ones steps, in evaluation to cities that completed steps late or in any manner.

Deadly Second Tide

The wave of the 1918 pandemic changed into extra lethal as compared to first. The wave had resembled flu epidemics; human beings most in risk had been older and the ill, while more in shape humans recovered. From August, once the second one wave started out in Sierra Leone France and the usa, the virus had mutated proper into a form. October 1918 become the month with the maximum fatality fee of the pandemic in its entirety. This seriousness changed into credited to the situations of the First World War. In lifestyles, a pressure is desired thru herbal preference. From the trench's desire emerge as reversed. Where they were infantrymen with a strain remained, on the equal time due to the fact the ill have been sent to vicinity hospitals to trains, dispersing the greater deadly virus. The 2d wave began, and the entire international changed into unfold at some stage in via way of using the influenza. Thus, in some unspecified time in the future of present day-day pandemics, fitness officials pay interest as quickly due to the fact the virus reaches regions with societal upheaval (searching out deadlier strains of this virus). The smooth truth that the majority of folks that recovered from ailments that were first-wave had turn out to be immune found out that it has to have been the pressure of influenza. This come to be dramatically exemplified in Copenhagen, which escaped the use of a joint mortality rate of just zero.29percent (zero.02 percent in the preliminary wave and zero.27 percent in the next wave) because of vulnerability to the lots much less-lethal first tide. For the ultimate part of the population, the subsequent wave have turn out to be loads greater mortal; the people that had been most exposed have been the ones together with the squaddies in the trenches -- adults that had been wholesome and younger.

Devastated Communities

Mass graves were dug via steam shovel and our bodies buried with out coffins in masses of regions. Pacific island lands had been hit difficult. The pandemic reached them from New Zealand, which have been sluggish to execute measures to stop from leaving its vents, boats, similar to the SS Talune, taking the flu. By New Zealand, the influenza attained Tonga (murdering eight percent of the populace), Nauru (16 percent), and Fiji

(5 percent, 9,000 people). Worst changed into Western Samoa German Samoa that changed into inhabited via New Zealand in 1914. Ninety percent of the population become inflamed; 22 percent of women 30 percent of men, and 10 percent of kids died. By assessment, the flu modified into prevented by the usage of using Governor John Martin Poyer with the resource of a blockade from achieving American Samoa. The disease unfold fastest via the social organizations some of the peoples, because of the addiction of gathering history from chiefs of their deathbed's network elders have been inflamed thru this machine. In New Zealand, 8,573 deaths were attributed to the 1918 pandemic flu, leading to an entire population fatality fee of zero.7 percentage. Māori were 8 to ten instances a good buy much less in all likelihood to die as Pakeha, because of the comparative poverty, more crowded domestic, rural population and lesser resistance to

infection. In 1918, the influenza accounted for 10 percent of the deaths in Ireland.

Less-Affected Places

China could in all likelihood have passed thru a slight flu season in 1918 in comparison to different regions of the planet. There changed into no organisation of health facts within the u . S . Within the period in-between, and a few reports out of its inner suggest that mortality costs from flu were more in at the least some locations in China. At the minimal, there may be minimum proof that the influenza affected China as an entire in evaluation to different international locations in the world. Though information from the indoors of China are missing, there has been statistics indexed in, like Harbin, Canton, Peking, Hong Kong and Shanghai. The Chinese Maritime Customs Service that has been staffed by manner of using foreigners, similar to the British, French, and extraordinary colonial officials in China accumulated this information. As a whole, low mortality prices are proven thru manner of actual information from the port cities of China in comparison to special towns in Asia. For example, the British government at Hong Kong and Canton said a mortality fee from flu at a tempo of 0.25 and zero.32 percentage, significantly decrease than the said mortality charge of different towns in Asia, for instance Calcutta or Bombay, at which flu changed into plenty extra catastrophic. From Shanghai's town -- that had a populace of extra than 2 million that there were simplest 266 deaths from flu some of the people in 1918. If extrapolated inside the big facts listed from Chinese towns, the proposed mortality fee from flu in China as a whole in 1918 have become likely lower than 1 percent -- drastically decrease than the area not unusual (that was about three--five percentage). By evaluation, Japan and Taiwan had stated a mortality rate from flu round zero.45% and zero.Sixty 9% respectively, extra than the mortality rate amassed from facts in Chinese port cities, which embody Hong Kong (zero.25 percent), Canton (0.32 percentage), and Shanghai. Back in Japan, 257,363 deaths had been attributed to the flu thru July 1919, presenting an predicted 0.4 percent mortality charge, which grow to be significantly decrease than nearly all distinctive Asian international places for which statistics are truely to be had. When the pandemic struck, the authorities constrained sea journeying to and from.

In American Samoa, the Pacific and the colony of New Caledonia succeeded in preventing a unmarried loss of existence thru quarantines. Almost 12,000 expired. From the notion of the island of Marajó, the pandemic in Brazil's Amazon River Delta hadn't stated an epidemic. No deaths were stated through Saint Helena. The passing despite the fact that the epidemiologists that toll in Russia modified into predicted at 450,000. If it's far proper, Russia out of place percent of its population -- the lowest mortality in Asia. This is considered via another check. The infrastructure of existence had damaged down Death toll changed into inside the direction of two percentage, or 2.7 million humans.

Aspirin Poisoning

In 2009, a paper discovered in the magazine Clinical Infectious Karen Starko recommended that aspirin poisoning contributed to the deaths. She based totally that at the said signs and symptoms and signs and symptoms and signs of people dying from the flu, as stated from the publish mortem critiques nevertheless to be had, similarly to the timing of this large "departure spike" in October 1918. This took place unexpectedly after the Surgeon General of the U.S. Army, together with the Journal of the American Medical Association, every advocated pretty massive doses of two to 31 grams of aspirin each day as a part of remedy. These portions created hyperventilation in lung edema in three percentage of patients, further to 33 percent of sufferers. Starko moreover notes that plenty of premature deaths tested "moist," now and again hemorrhagic lungs, even as overdue deaths determined bacterial pneumonia. She indicates that the tide of aspirin poisonings grow to be the give up result of a "awesome typhoon" of activities: Bayer's patent on aspirin died, such a number of companies rushed in to earn a gain and extensively superior the supply; this collaborated with the Spanish influenza; and the symptoms and symptoms of aspirin poisoning have been no longer acknowledged within the intervening time. For instance, for its immoderate mortality fee, this idea modified into contested in a letter to the magazine discovered in April 2010 through Andrew Noymer and Daisy Carreon of the University of California, Irvine, and Niall Johnson of the Australian Commission on Safety and Quality in Healthcare. They contested the applicability of this aspirin idea, for the cause that the excessive mortality fee in which there was no or little access to aspirin inside the 2nd, in evaluation to the loss of life rate in areas. They reasoned that "the salicylate aspirin poisoning precept turned into difficult to maintain because the maximum critical motive for the unusual virulence of the 1918-1919 flu pandemic." In response, Starko stated there has been clinical evidence of aspirin utilization in India and contended that if aspirin over-prescription hadn't contributed to the extended Indian mortality charge, it would despite the fact that manifest to be a element for increased charges in places in which special exacerbating elements decided in India executed a feature.

Chapter 3: What's Spanish Flu?

This influenza is likewise referred to as the 1918 influenza pandemic, or the lethal flu. Lasting from January 1918 500 million human beings -- shape of a third of the planet's populace – had been inflamed with the beneficial useful resource of it. The death toll was predicted to have been everywhere from as big as one hundred million, and 17 million to 50 million, which makes it the numerous deadliest pandemics in facts. World War I censored faded opinions of mortality and contamination inside the USA, the United Kingdom, France, and Germany to preserve sanity. Newspapers had been unfastened to file the epidemic's results in neutral Spain, similar to the grave infection of King Alfonso XIII, and such recollections generated a faux perception of Spain as mainly hard hit. This gave upward thrust. Ancient and epidemiological statistics are inadequate to pick out with truth that the pandemics geographical supply, with diverse perspectives concerning its place. Most flu outbreaks kill the very more youthful and the very antique, the usage of a more survival fee for all of the ones in among, but the Spanish influenza pandemic prompted a greater than anticipated mortality rate for adults. Researchers provide severa motives for its excessive mortality price of the 1918 flu pandemic. Some investigations have established the virus to be mainly deadly because it activates a cytokine typhoon, which ravages the greater effective immune device of young adults. By evaluation, a 2007 assessment of fitness care journals within the period of the pandemic determined that the viral sickness modified into now not any more competitive than previous flu lines. Rather, hygiene, overcrowded spas and hospitals, and malnourishment endorsed contamination. This infection changed into deadly to all sufferers. The Spanish influenza modified into the number one of two pandemics because of the flu virus; the subsequent have end up that influenza in 2009.

What's The Flu?

Influenza, or flu, is an endemic that attacks the breathing machine. The influenza virus is quite infectious: If an inflamed man or woman coughs, sneezes or talks, respiration droplets are created and transmitted to the surroundings, and can be inhaled via all and sundry close to. Furthermore, someone who rolls some issue with the whole virus onto it and then touches their mouth, nostril, or eyes might also additionally furthermore get inflamed. Flu outbreaks arise every year and alternate in severity, depending in component on which kind of virus is spreading. (Flu viruses can fast mutate.)

Spanish Influenza: The Virus That Changed The World

A sickness commenced to comb a deadly virus that inflamed a 3rd of the planet's population and left upwards of fifty million useless. Laura Spinney investigated the devastating impact of the Spanish influenza pandemic and the manner it contrasted the Coronavirus catastrophe on 28 September 1918. A Spanish paper gave its traffic a brief lesson on flu. "The representative responsible for this illness, it's far your Pfeiffer's bacillus, which can be very tiny and observable pleasant by way of a microscope." The clarification become because of the truth the complete international come to be in the draw close to in their very barbarous influenza pandemic on document -- however it modified into wrong: influenza is due to an epidemic. The concept that influenza become because of a bacillus or Illness turned into authorized with the useful resource of the most notable scientists of their day, who'd discover themselves almost clearly helpless within the face of the scourge.

Just How Many People Died From The Spanish Flu?

Spanish influenza became a few of the deadliest failures in statistics. It lasted for 2 a long term -- the various earliest documented example in March 1918 and the past in March 1920, an estimated 50 million human beings died, regardless of the fact that a few specialists indicate that the whole might have been double. Even the 'Spanish flu' murdered at some point of the First World War, possibly more than the Second World War.

How Can Spanish Influenza Compare To Coronavirus?Laura Spinney cautioned me "You may additionally moreover have located a decide floating about of a case fatality price of three.Four percentage, which describes the ratio of people who seize the COVID-19 illness who go to die of it. The quantity that is regularly quoted for its Spanish Flu, as an example, the case fatality charge is .5percent however it's miles a completely, very, very arguable parent for the purpose that quantities are so hard to understand. I suggest we don't forget that probably 50 million human beings died but there wasn't any shape of dependable test in the time absolutely so we cannot be satisfied about that which super cries all of the numbers out." So, it's miles in reality hard to create the historic comparisons, even within the event which you've had been given correct statistics in recent times, which we do not. Therefore, on both facet of the equation, even in case you pick, it's far a transferring target. "We'd glaringly like to get a vaccine from COVID-19 nowadays but we do no longer and we would want to wait a 12 months to 18 months because of that. They'd have no vaccine in any respect in 1918. Or as a substitute they did create molds however they have been unworthy, quite a bargain, as they have been essentially pathogens in the direction of bacteria inside the respiratory tract while, as we recognize, influenza is a viral infection. So, concerning this, we're advanced in evaluation to 1918. But we do not have that vaccine. We have anti-inflammatory remedy for treating the sick and we have got antibiotics with a purpose to be useful for treating the bacterial ailments that might cause pneumonia once in a while, as they did in 1918, reputedly."

The pandemic struck in a vital juncture of comprehension of infection that is infectious. Well into the nineteenth century, epidemics were taken into consideration acts of God -- a perception that dated again into the Middle Ages. Originally, even though compounds had been positioned within the 17th century, they had been no longer related with issues. In the 1850s, the French biologist Louis Pasteur made the hyperlink among contamination and micro-organisms, and by using using manner of more than one microbiologist Robert Koch furthered notions of contamination. 'Germ idea' turn out to be disseminated a long way and huge, converting thoughts that have been fatalistic. The 20th century, together with improvements in sanitation and hygiene, had made massive inroads from the so-called 'target market' ailments that affected human businesses, in particular those inhabiting the great cities which had mushroomed inside the aftermath of the monetary revolution. Through the nineteenth century many urbanites had been dropped to illnesses -- cholera, tuberculosis, and typhus, to mention 3 -- which cities had a non-prevent inflow of peasants inside the geographical vicinity to maintain their numbers up. At remaining that that that they had end up self-explanatory.

Where Did The Spanish Flu Originate?Some theories advocate it did now not start in Spain. We do not recognize in which it commenced, but we realize it did not start in Spain. The Spanish had been, to a point, stigmatized with this. Even even though the trenches of the First World War are nevertheless a contender, there is moreover no manner of being positive in which Spanish Flu originated. The soldiers' immune system modified. It's believed earlier than spreading at an alarming tempo to Europe, the instances had been the pandemic modified into called 'Spanish Flu.' Censorship exaggerated the consequences of the virus in Spain. While Britain, France, Germany, and the united states censored and constrained early reviews, newspapers in Spain -- as a unbiased state -- have been liberated to talk all of the dreadful information of this pandemic.

From 1918, religion in mathematics become low, and large scientists had followed a swagger. Twenty years before, this had inspired the Irish playwright George Bernard Shaw to compose the medical doctor's Dilemma, in which an eminent health practitioner, Sir Colenso Ridgeon -- a person steady with Sir Almroth Wright, who developed the typhoid vaccine -- performs god collectively together with his patients' destinies. Shaw changed into warning physicians toward hubris; however, it required an endemic of some different 'audience' sickness -- flu -- to hold them home they understood. When scientists believed approximately 'germs' from the 20th century, they concept approximately germs. The virus have become a completely unique precept; its capability had inflamed tobacco flowers and located the virus, decided in 1892. Unlike germs, it have been too little to be considered via an optical microscope. Without having simply decided viruses, scientists mimicked their individual. They were veiled in thriller, and no man or woman guessed that they is probably the reason for the flu. Throughout the influenza pandemic -- the so-called 'Russian' flu, which began out in 1889 -- a pupil of Koch's known as Richard Pfeiffer promised to have identified. Pfeiffer's bacillus, as it have been recognized, can cause infection and does exist -- however it would not reason flu. During the 1918 pandemic, pathologists who cultivated bacterial colonies inside the lung tissue of influenza patients determined Pfeiffer's bacillus in positive, however not all of the civilizations, which harassed them. To upload to physicians' puzzlement, vaccines generated from the bacillus of Pfeiffer seemed to advantage some patients. Actually, those experiments have been successful toward secondary bacterial illnesses that triggered pneumonia -- that the first-rate purpose of dying in most instances -- however scientists did no longer understand that in the inside the interim. They'd recognise that it modified right into a mistake.

Flu Season

In the usa, "flu season" usually runs from late Fall into spring. In a regular yr, over hundred,000 Americans are hospitalized for flu-associated headaches, and within the remaining 3 a long time, there were numerous 3,000 to 49,000 flu-related U.S. Deaths every 12 months, consistent with the Centers for Disease Control and Prevention. Young youngsters, individuals over age sixty 5, pregnant ladies, and those with unique clinical conditions, like diabetes, bronchial bronchial asthma, or cardiovascular sickness, face a extra chance of flu-related headaches, consisting of pneumonia, sinus, ear infections and hepatitis. Influenza pandemic, similar to the only in 1918, occurs whilst a specially virulent new flu strain for which there may be little if any immunity arises and spreads unexpectedly from individual to person across the area.

Spanish Flu Symptoms

The initial wave of the 1918 pandemic befell inside the spring and have become slight. The unwell, which underwent such commonplace influenza symptoms like chills, fatigue, and fever, commonly recovered after some days, and furthermore the form of said deaths changed into decreased. The 2nd wave of flu appeared in the autumn of that 12 months with a vengeance. Victims died inner days or hours of signs and symptoms and signs and symptoms. By a couple of years, the not unusual lifestyles expectancy in America dropped 1918, in 1 twelve months.

What Led To The Spanish Flu?

It is unknown exactly in which the precise breed of Flu that delivered at the pandemic originated. Nonetheless, the 1918 influenza end up first detected in Europe, America, and regions of Asia earlier than spreading to almost each distinct a part of the area in a keep in mind of weeks. Regardless of the reality that the 1918 influenza emerge as no longer isolated to a place, it have become famous spherical the region due to the truth that Spanish influenza, Spain changed into struck tough by using the contamination and wasn't situation to the malevolent news blackouts that affected extraordinary European international places. (Spain's king, Alfonso XIII, allegedly contracted the flu) 1 ordinary factor of the 1918 influenza turn out to be that it struck many formerly wholesome, more youthful human beings – a band generally resistant to this shape of infectious sickness – including loads of World War I servicemen. In fact, many more U.S. Infantrymen died from the 1918 influenza than were killed within the warfare at some degree inside the conflict. Forty percentage of the U.S. Navy changed into struck with the flu, at the identical time as 36% of the Army have become unwell. Soldiers moving throughout the planet in crowded trains and ships helped to disperse the killer virus. Additional estimates run as large as 3% of the planet's population. The loss of life toll attributed to the influenza is expected at 20 million to 50 million sufferers globally. The numbers aren't possible to apprehend because of a deficiency of health. What is known is that locations have been evidence towards the 1918 influenza – to human beings of communities which have been a long manner flung, patients ranged from citizens of towns in America. Even President Woodrow Wilson allegedly gotten smaller influenza in early 1919 whilst negotiating the Treaty of Versailles, which ended World War I.

Why Was The Spanish Flu Called Spanish?

The Spanish Flu did now not get up in Spain. Spain have grow to be a country with a press that included the outbreak in Madrid in May from the begin. Meanwhile, the Central Powers, in addition to Allied countries, had censors who protected statistics of this influenza up to preserve morale immoderate. Since Spanish data property had been now not the simplest ones reporting on influenza, many considered it originated there (the Spanish, in the meantime, considered the virus originated out of France and referred to as it the "French Flu.")

Where Did The Spanish Flu Come From?

Scientists do not understand for nice in which the Flu originated. Concepts point to France, China, Britain, and moreover america, in which the earliest example have come to be stated on March 11, 1918, in Camp Funston at Fort Riley, Kansas. Some recall squaddies that had been infected had unfold the contamination in some unspecified time in the destiny of the nation to navy camps. In March 1918, the subsequent month squaddies led throughout the Atlantic and have been determined carefully thru 118,000 greater.

First Instances Reported From The Deadly Spanish Influenza Pandemic

Before breakfast at the afternoon of March four, Albert Mitchell of the U.S. Army reviews on the hospital in Fort Riley, Kansas, whining of these cold-like symptoms of sore throat, ache, and fever. By evaluation, over one hundred of his fellow soldiers had suggested symptoms and signs that were comparable, signaling what are concept to be the initial instances from the flu pandemic of 1918. Influenza would kill an envisioned 20 million to 50 million people and 675,000 Americans the world over, proving to be a far extra deadly force than the First World War. The outbreak of this disease has been found with the resource of outbreaks in prisons and army camps in pretty a few areas of the usa. The disorder all of sudden traveled to Europe together with the American infantrymen going to assist the Allies in the battlefields of France (Back in March 1918 by myself, eighty four,000 American soldiers led for the duration of the Atlantic; but each different 118,000 positioned them some other month). Influenza observed no symptoms and signs and symptoms of abating at the identical time as it came on some specific continent: 31,000 instances were stated in

Great Britain in June. The sickness become speedy dubbed Spanish influenza because of a quite better variety of deaths in Spain (a few 8 million, it were said) following the primary outbreak there in May 1918. No mercy become showed thru influenza on every side of the trenches for combatants. The preliminary wave of the outbreak hit closer to German forces, wherein they waged a remaining offensive that could set up the consequences of the warfare. It had a large effect at the morale in their troops due to the fact the flu deepened losses, along side terrible provisions depressing the spirits of fellows in the III Infantry Division. The flu unfold past the boundaries of Western Europe. The close of the summer time had instances suggested in Russia, North Africa, and India; New Zealand, Japan, the Philippines similarly to China might fall victim. The Great War ended on November eleven, however flu endured to wreak worldwide havoc, flaring another time inside the U.S. Within a greater vicious wave together with the flow decrease back of infantrymen in the direction of the warfare and ultimately infecting an expected 28 percentage of the nation's population earlier than it in the end petered out.

Fighting The Spanish Flu

Scientists and clinical doctors were uncertain after the 1918 flu strike what added on it or how to attend to it. There have been pills which handled the flu but no vaccines or antivirals. (The first actual legal flu vaccine emerged in America in the 1940s. By the following decade, vaccine makers can also need to routinely create vaccines that would assist restrain and shield towards potential pandemics). Complicating topics was the reality that World War I had deserted a loss of scientific medical doctors and one of a kind medical examiners to quantities of America. And of that available clinical personnel from the U.S., many came again with the flu themselves. Hospitals in awesome regions have been bombarded with influenza patients who unique homes, non-public houses, and faculties had to be transformed to hospitals, a number of which have been staffed with students. Officials in superb regions imposed quarantines at the side of church houses, schools, and theaters. People have been encouraged furthermore to stay inner and also to keep away from shaking arms, libraries located a block on regulations and financing books. According to the New York Times, in some unspecified time in the future of the ordeal, Boy Scouts in New York approached human beings that that they had seen spitting on the road and gave them playing playing cards which look at: "You're in violation of this Sanitary Code."

Aspirin Poisoning And The Flu

Without remedy for the flu physicians, they believed it'd relieve signs and symptoms. For instance: aspirin, which changed into trademarked via the use of Bayer in 1899 –

a patent which died in 1917, that means easy businesses might also want to create the drugs in a few unspecified time inside the destiny of the Spanish Flu outbreak. Prior to the spike in deaths attributed to the Spanish Flu in 1918, the U.S. Surgeon General, Navy and moreover the Journal of the American Medical Association had advocated using aspirin. Medical experts advised sufferers to take round 30g each day. (For evaluation's sake, the health consensus now might be that doses over 4g is volatile). Indicators of aspirin poisoning embody the buildup of fluid inside the lungs, or hyperventilation, and edema, and it believed that some of hastened or of those October deaths have been because of aspirin poisoning.

The Flu Takes Heavy Toll On Society

Influenza took infinite lives; developing widows and orphans. Funeral parlors have been full of our bodies as they commenced piling up. People had to dig graves for his or her very very very own Relatives. The influenza changed into injurious to the market. From america, due to the fact many personnel said they were pressured to shut down ill. Basic offerings like trash series and mail delivery had been hindered due to employees. There had been farm employees to harvest plant life. Even community and state health departments close down for corporation, hampering tries to supply and to chronicle the unfold of the 1918 influenza People approximately it with responses.

The Way U.S. Cities Try To Stop The 1918 Flu Pandemic

A catastrophic tide of the Spanish Flu struck American beaches inside the summer time of 1918 and unfold to severa cities. With no vaccine or remedy application, it dropped to officers and mayors to improvise plans to defend the residents. With pressure to seem patriotic at wartime and with a censored media downplaying the disorder's unfold, many made tragic alternatives. The manner to Philadelphia changed into too little, too overdue. Dr. Wilmer Krusen, manager of Public Health and Charities for the town, insisted mounting deaths have been no longer the "Spanish flu," however as an possibility the pleasant influenza. The city moved with a Liberty Loan parade spreading the infection. More than 1,000 Philadelphians have been useless. Only then did the city near saloons and theaters. From March 1919, their private lives had been misplaced through over 15,000 residents of Philadelphia. St. Louis, Missouri, changed into outstanding: Schools and film theaters closed and public events had been prohibited. As a result, the peak mortality fee in St. Louis turn out to be only one-eighth of Philadelphia's passing price in some unspecified time in the future of the height of the outbreak. Citizens at San Francisco were fined $5 when they were stuck with out a masks and charged with worrying the peace.

Spanish Flu Pandemic Ends

From the summer of 1919, the influenza pandemic got here to an end; folks that were inflamed every acquired resistance or expired. Nearly ninety a few years after, in 2008, researchers delivered that they had determined precisely what made the 1918 flu so lethal: A bunch of 3 genes allowed the virus to weaken a victim's bronchial tubes and lungs and easy the way for bacterial pneumonia. Too lethal, there have been different flu pandemics thinking about that 1918. An influenza pandemic from 1957 to 1958 killed round million humans globally, together with some 70,000 people in America, along component furthermore an epidemic from 1968 to 1969 killed about 1 million human beings, along facet some 34,000 Americans. Over 12,000 Americans expired at some point of the H1N1 (or “swine flu") pandemic, which occurred from 2009 to 2010. The novel covid outbreak of 2020 is spreading round the world as nations race to find a remedy for COVID 19 and taxpayers safe haven installation that allows you to prevent spreading the illness, which can be very lethal because of the fact most carriers are asymptomatic for instances in advance than spotting they're inflamed. Every one of these modern-day-day pandemics brings renewed hobby in and interest on the Spanish Flu, or “forgotten pandemic," so-named even as you take into account that its spread had been overshadowed with the useful useful resource of the deadliness of both WWI and coated through way of information blackouts and insufficient report-keeping.

Chapter 4: Why Can It Be Known As 'Spanish Flu'?

Influenza had obtained its name as it had been perception to have originated from Bukhara in Uzbekistan (at the time, a part of the Russian empire). The pandemic, which broke out nearly 30 a long time after will continuously be referred to as the 'Spanish flu', even though it did not begin in Spain. It washed at some point of the complete global in three waves that, at the northern hemisphere, corresponded to a few gentle wave in the spring of 1918, a deadly wave the subsequent fall, and reprisal from the number one months of 1919, which changed into intermediate in virulence among each. The instances had been indexed at Camp Funston. Within six weeks that the infection had reached the trenches of the western the front in France, but, it become most effective in May that influenza broke out in Spain. Contrary to the us and France, Spain have become independent in the warfare; consequently it did not censor its own press. The first Spanish instances had been suggested inside the papers, additionally considering that King Alfonso XIII, the excessive minister, and masses of people of this cupboard have been this kind of early instances; the dominion's plight became rather observable. People spherical the arena concept that the disease had rippled from Madrid -- a false impression advocated through manner of propagandists inside the ones belligerent global places that knew that they had contracted it earlier than Spain. In the interest of retaining morale immoderate internal their populations, they were thrilled to trade the blame. The discover stuck. Understandably, Spaniards smarted at this calumny: they understood that they weren't responsible, and imagined the French of having sent influenza at some degree in the boundary, but they could not be glad. They throw around for some other tag, moreover located perception in an operetta executed in the capital Zarzuela

Theatre -- a specifically popular reworking of the myth of Don Juan, with a catchy tune called 'The Soldier of Naples'. The complex illness have become well-known in Spain because the 'Naples Soldier.' Although the Spanish flu did no longer begin in Spain that united states did undergo very badly with it. From the early twentieth century, influenza became appeared as a democratic contamination -- no one have become immune closer to it however, inside the thick of this pandemic, it had been noticed that the sickness struck. It 'favored' unique age instructions: the very younger and the older, however additionally a middle cohort elderly 20 to forty. It preferred guys to ladies, with the exclusion of pregnant women, who've been at mainly large risk. This age and gender-associated styles have been replicated all over the planet, but, the virulence with influenza struck severa from area to location. Inhabitants of particular factors of Asia had been a stunning 30 times much more likely to die from the flu than human beings in areas of Europe. Generally, Asia and Africa suffered maximum loss of life costs, collectively with the most inexpensive located in Europe, North America, and Australia. However, there has been great version in continents, additionally. African nations south of the Sahara professional demise speeds or maybe 3 instances more than the ones north of the barren region, even as Spain indexed a number of the maximum passing prices in Europe -- double that in Britain, 3 instances that in Denmark. The unevenness did now not save you there. Generally, towns persisted worse than rural places, however a few towns persisted worse than many others, and there was additionally variation in towns. Newly arrived immigrants tended to die extra often than older, better-set up corporations, for example. In the geographical location, one village might be decimated on the equal time as every distinct, apparently similar in each manner, were given away with a slight dose.

What Kinds Of People Caught The Spanish Flu?

Influenza regarded to attack with an detail of randomness and cruelty. Since adults in their top died in droves, unlucky businesses imploded. Kids had been orphaned, older dad and mom made to fend for them. Individuals have been at a loss to present an reason for this clean lottery, and it left them profoundly disturbed. Trying to make clear the sensation that it inspired in him, a French medical doctor in the city of Lyons wrote that it have been instead in evaluation to the “gut pangs" he'd skilled while serving at the the the the front. This has been "a extra deep stress, the feeling of a few indefinable terror which had taken hold of the people of the metropolis." It became first-rate in a while while epidemiologists zeroed in on the quantities that patterns started out out to emerge, and the preliminary elements of justification had been set ahead. A type of the variety can be defined through manner of manner of inequalities of wealth and caste -- and, to the amount, it represented the ones variables: pores and pores and skin color, awful weight loss plan, crowded living conditions, and confined get admission to to healthcare weakened the constitution, which makes the awful, immigrants, and cultural minorities extra vulnerable to disorder. As French historian Patrick Zylberman stated: “The virus may additionally moreover moreover have behaved ‘democratically,' however the manner of existence it assaulted became now and again egalitarian."

Any different underlying illness made a person greater prone to the Spanish flu, at the same time as preceding exposure to influenza itself modulates the seriousness of a state of affairs. Remote corporations with out masses historic revel in of this contamination suffered badly, as did cities which have been bypassed thru way of the primary wave of the pandemic because of the truth they have been not immunologically ‘primed’ to the second one. As an instance, Rio de Janeiro – the capital of Brazil on the time – received best one wave of flu in October 1918, and experienced a loss of existence fee or three times higher than that recorded in American towns to the north that had received every the spring and autumn waves. And Bristol Bay in Alaska became spared before early 1919, however if the virus ultimately obtained a foothold it decreased the bay Eskimo population through forty percentage. Public fitness efforts made a difference, irrespective of the fact that medics did not recognize the motive for the illness. Since time immemorial, if contagion is a danger human beings have practiced 'social distancing' -- information unconsciously that steerage clear of infected humans will growth the opportunity of staying healthful. Back in 1918, social distancing took the form of quarantine zones, isolation wards, and prohibitions on mass activities; in which they had been efficiently enforced, the ones steps slowed the unfold. Australia maintained out the autumn wave actually through imposing a a achievement quarantine in its ports. Exceptions confirmed the rule of thumb of thumb. Back in 1918, Persia modified into a collapsed u . S . After a long time of getting used as a pawn within the 'Great Game' -- that the war the numerous British and the Russians for control of this big place between the Arabian and Caspian Seas. Its authorities turn out to be inclined and nearly broke, and it lacked a coherent sanitary infrastructure. Therefore, every time the flu diminished from the northeastern holy metropolis of Mashhad in August 1918, no social distancing measures had been enforced. In a fortnight every house and administrative center from Mashhad have been infected, and additionally -thirds of this metropolis's population fell ill that autumn. With no boundaries on motion, influenza spread thickly with pilgrims, infantrymen, and shops to the four corners of the united states of the us. From now Persia emerge as freed from influenza, it had dropped amongst eight% and 22 percent of its personal population (that doubt representing the truth that, in a country in disaster, accumulating records changed into slightly a challenge). Even eight percentage equates to the mortality charge in Ireland.

Where disparities in costs of infection and death had been perceived, humans's reasons pondered cutting-edge statistics – or, as an alternative, misunderstanding – of infectious contamination. When Charles Darwin laid out his principle of evolution via natural desire in On the Origin of Species (1859), he had no longer intended his mind to be carried out to human societies, but others of his time did just that, growing the 'generation' of eugenics. Eugenicists believed that mankind blanketed 'races' and from 1918 their thinking changed into mainstream. Some eugenicists observed that sectors of society suffered towards influenza, which they credited to a few inferiority. They'd included germ concept in their global angle: on the same time because the terrible and the running instructions have been prone to ailment, concluded the eugenicists, they only had themselves accountable, because of the reality Pasteur had advised that illness changed into preventable.

Indian Anxieties

The outcomes of the road of questioning are exemplified in India. That land's British colonizers had lengthy taken the view that India grow to be inherently unhygienic, and so had invested little in indigenous healthcare. As many as 18 million Indians died within the pandemic -- that the good deal in numbers of any state on the earth. However, there was a backlash. Resentment modified into fueled through the British reply to the unfold of influenza. Tensions came to a head with the passage in 1919. This caused calm protests, and on 13 April British troops fired into an unarmed crowd in Amritsar, murdering countless Indian human beings -- a bloodbath that galvanized the liberty motion. Uprisings were delivered approximately through the usage of influenza some location else. The fall of 1918 observed a tide of employees' actions and protests round the sector. Disgruntlement became smoldering due to the fact that preceding to the Russian revolutions of 1917, but influenza fanned the flames by manner of exacerbating what became a dire deliver state of affairs, moreover via highlighting inequality. Even well-ordered Switzerland narrowly prevented a civil struggle in November 1918 following leftwing organizations attributed to a large type of influenza deaths from the army on the government and military control. There have been areas of the planet wherein people hadn't heard of Darwin or germ precept, and in which the human beings end up reasons which are more tried-and-examined. From the agricultural interior of China, as an example, an entire lot of people notwithstanding the reality that idea that contamination had been despatched by way of using dragons and demons; they paraded amounts of dinosaurs through the roads within the choice of appeasing the irate spirits. A missionary scientific physician described going from house to residence in Shanxi province in early 1919, and locating scissors positioned indoors "to keep off demons or constant with chance to reduce them in 2". In the west that was modernized, people vacillated lack of existence regularly regarded to strike without rhyme or cause. Many though remembered a more mystical, pre-Darwinian generation, and 4 years of conflict had worn down intellectual defenses. Seeing how their guys of era were to assist them, most people got here to anticipate that the stunt become an act of god retribution because of their sins. In Zamora -- precisely the precise identical Spanish metropolis whose paper said with such self guarantee the representative of illness were Pfeiffer's bacillus -- that the bishop defied the fitness government' ban on mass activities and ordered people to the dinosaurs to placate "God's legitimate anger." This city then recorded some of the maximum demise tolls from influenza in Spain -- a easy fact of which its population have been conscious, regardless of the truth that they do no longer seem to have held it from their personal bishop. They gave him a trophy in recognition of his tries to surrender his or her suffering. This illustrates gulfs were represented with the useful aid of solutions to influenza.

Chapter 5: Impacts Of The Spanish Flu At The American Nation

In the autumn of 1918, the area peace taken away through the Great War in Europe come to be again at the horizon. The conflict changed into winding down despite the fact that the U.S. Had joined forces months in advance just so Allied Forces is probably helped to complete routing out Germany. The troops contributed via America were uncovered to the worst situations of life deep in the trenches.

In the final three hundred and sixty five days of World War 1, an influenza A virus called H1N1 broke out. Though it turn out to be named the Spanish flu for wrong reasons, the number one times on record happened in the United States in March of the very last one year of the Great War.

How Spanish Flu Began in America

Some critics have opined that America's, therefore the area's, Spanish influenza case won't be as horrible if America's troops have been better cared for. Well, all of us is entitled to his opinion. However, there may be a few elements of truth in that complaint thinking about how the flu impacted the usa and Americans.

Consider the chronicle in keeping with the e-book The Great Influenza. The 2005 book described a community physician Loring Miner experience. Miner located the ordeal of a few people, 1720 of them, inside the cautiously populated county occupying 578 rectangular miles. At some issue, the strong and healthy humans have been certainly coming down with a surprisingly violent stress of flu.

Concerned through the usage of what he noticed, Miner notified the U.S. Public Health Service in 1918 and sounded the warning about a brand new form of flu. But with the beneficial resource of March 1918, the sickness appeared to have burned itself out. The struggle pastimes gave a faux guarantee that the flu won't spread beyond Haskell County. So the struggle endured as ordinary and people have been shifting inside and outside of America and round america of the usa more than ever.

Military Camp Funston

Even more youthful men from the county training nearby at Camp Funston (now Fort Riley, Kansas) had loose motion from their homes to the camp and again. The from side to side persevered even though on go away. While Dr. Miner became searching for to determine the reason of peculiar deaths some of the citizens of Haskell County within the spring of 1918, the network boys had been unperturbed, in step with the community paper, as they overtly moved to and from Camp Funston.

By the middle of March 1918, 48 of those troops at Fort Riley died of pneumonia due to the flu, regardless of the fact that the purpose changed into now not ascertained.

Many infected infantrymen from Fort Riley have been nonetheless sent to Europe. Back there in Europe, the virus mutated due to the truth the infected American squaddies interacted with English, French, and German soldiers. The mutation have come to be greater lethal and the returnee American infantrymen introduced the flu with them.

About that time, over one hundred thirty,000 out of the 1.2 million American infantrymen were hospitalized with this identical flu. And a huge percentage of them didn't come decrease returned alive. Toward the give up of 1918, no longer less than 45,000 soldiers from America have been killed, not via the enemies' bullet, but thru influenza and associated pneumonia. That changed into somewhere among one-location and one-1/three of American infantrymen killed in four years thru the struggle.

Experiences of Camps Devens

That identical month, the virulent strain of the influenza virus seemed at Camp Devens in Massachusetts. Out of the 50,000 population of the camp, 14,000 were down with the flu. The Army determined to quarantine the camp. So they sent a contingent of the troop to Camp Upton on Long Island close to Yaphank. 757 infantrymen had been out of place to the same foe.

The then appearing Surgeon General of the U.S. Army, Victor Vaughn, have turn out to be ordered to immediately file to Camp Devens near Boston to move and check the scenario. What he noticed bowled over him. Hear his firsthand account: "I determined hundreds of extra younger stalwart men in uniform moving into the wards of the hospital. Every bed have become whole, but others crowded in. The faces wore a bluish robust; a cough introduced up the blood-stained sputum. In the morning, the lifeless our bodies are stacked approximately the morgue like cordwood." Influenza felled sixty 3 squaddies that day in September 1918.

And in Camp Upton

The a protracted manner off Camp Upton didn't fare pretty in a unique manner. It grow to be the meeting region of the National Guard's 40 second Division. It have grow to be additionally the education camp for the 77th Division, specifically the draftees from New York City. The Spanish flu paid the 40 three,000 thousand navy population and an ugly visit on September 13. Four days later (September 17), 171 of them had been hospitalized.

The only proactive (albeit retroactive) steps Colonel John S. Mallory in charge of the camp may also need to take were shutting down the camp to civilian web site site visitors and finishing leaves for the troops. Defending his motion at the equal time as asked by way of the usage of the New York

Times, Mallory said he had to that to avoid the spread of the sickness stressing that no matter the reality that, there were no deaths in Camp Upton, he must prevent the camp from being badly hit.

But by means of the usage of the stop of that month, three,050 cases of Spanish influenza were said at Camp Upton. 401 infantrymen inside the camp were stricken by pneumonia. Eventually, the camp out of place 15 infantrymen to the flu on October 1, 1918. The virus outbreak at Camp Upton didn't give up there. It reached its pinnacle on October four, 1918. According to one of the evaluations made with the resource of the use of the military base medical institution commander, the virus sent 483 squaddies had been to the health facility on October five.

That delivered the whole substantial shape of showed times within the camp to 4,371. That day, influenza killed 20 of them. Stricter measures have been taken to prevent the unfold and prevent similarly infection. The New York Times reviews that soldiers had been ordered to place on gauze mask, which include: "Soldiers will now not be accredited to take a seat down opposite each one-of-a-kind at mess tables. Foodstuffs other than in sealed programs will no longer be offered in the placed up exchanges, and no individual unmasked can be authorised in any YMCA or different welfare constructing."

Civilian Fatality

Meanwhile, due to the strict wartime media censorship within the warring nations, there was silence conspiracy concerning what was going on at the battlefields and navy camps. No information modified into reporting this to warn the civilian populace of what become step by step becoming an epidemic.

Civilians near army camps had been freely stepping into and out of those camps as they had been unaware of the deadly infection. Some of them who have been observant enough to see unwell infantrymen attributed their condition to conflict fatigue or some ugly evaluations from the the front. They had been going about visiting or doing their everyday business organization with them.

These civilian populations have been contracting this ailment and were taking it home to others. And that the civilians had been now not underneath routine; that they had more freedom of motion. Consequently, they helped spread influenza among communities. It took a while earlier than they found out what have emerge as happening.

It changed into in May 1918 whilst Spain officially added it and commenced out giving it wider insurance that the American public fitness officials issued a warning about an coming near near (but in truth already ravaging) flu they referred to as the

“Spanish influenza”. Before then, the harm were done.

The disorder took greater lives among civilians than amongst infantrymen that have been believed to introduce it. Eventually, Spanish influenza claimed the lives of about 675,000 Americans in 1918 by myself. That have turn out to be hundreds extra than the form of Americans killed at a few level inside the conflict, given at lots much less than two hundred,000.

Other strata of American society had a awesome nasty ordeal with the flu. What efforts were made to comprise it? The American Spanish flu story maintains.

Chapter 6: Dealing With The Scourge The American Way

The pandemic affected each person physically or emotionally. One-area of the American population had been infected with influenza. It modified into almost not feasible to be absolutely loose. There have grow to be palpable fear among people who hadn't shriveled it. They didn't recognize even as and the manner they might be infected.

Even the warmongering President Woodrow Wilson wasn't spared. During the negotiations for the vital treaty of Versailles in a bid to hold the struggle to an stop, he reportedly shrunk the flu. Those who control or were fortunate enough no longer to be infected had their social lives critically altered via manner of the general public health ordinances issued to cut back the unfold of influenza or the priority of unknown.

Shortage of Medical Personnel and Facility

The World War complicated America's case with the Spanish flu in numerous different techniques. Take the case of Camp Syracuse as an instance. In August, there were remoted times. But on September 4, 10,000 new draftees arrived from Massachusetts to the camp that changed into not a eternal facility. Soldiers have been dwelling carefully together in overcrowded tents.

Since there has been no sanatorium inside the camp, sick soldiers had been noted civilian hospitals in Fort Ontario or Syracuse. Before quick hospitals had been built, the camp changed into already overfilled with four hundred sufferers and a 3rd of the forty clinical employees there have been added down via the virus. As the unwell squaddies have been being sent to civilian hospitals, the illness have become spreading short in the most vital Syracuse. This resulted within the lack of life of 900 residents and 208 soldiers camping nearby.

Many of America's physicians were either attending to the war victims or were down with influenza themselves. So there was an acute shortage of medical examiners normally. Medical centers had been stretched to the restriction a lot so that infirmaries in sure regions were overloaded with flu sufferers. Schools, church homes, and different homes which incorporates non-public homes had to be transformed into makeshift scientific centers. Even then, those were staffed high-quality by means of clinical college students.

Sending More to Their Ruin

The call for for more troops didn’t assist the problem. Doctors of the American Expeditionary Force in Europe were treating 340,000 hospitalized infantrymen who had been down with influenza in 1918 on the same time as some other 227,000 troops have been moreover hospitalized for injuries sustained in struggle. Still, there was a name for brought squaddies.

In October 1918, due to the truth the U.S. American Army inside the offensive at Meuse-Argonne, they were locked in battle, pushing with efficiently within the path of the Germans. 1,451 Americans died from the flu. The large sort of 1/3 Infantry Division Soldiers evacuated from the battlefront due to influenza is extra than that of these injured in fight.

All the machine for drafting and schooling new soldiers had been close down because of the epidemic. America is now at the crux: German troops were retreating, however the U.S. Squaddies were being killed and wounded. The commander of the AEF, Gen. John J. Pershing, demanded reinforcements. According to Army Surgeon General Charles Richard, but, it wasn't expedient to deliver more infantrymen to France till the epidemic stopped.

But President Woodrow Wilson didn't count on so. In his view, inside the occasion that they stopped the reinforcement now,

Germans could probable have respiration room to rejig their method. So the Army Chief of Staff Payton March due despatched the troop to exigencies. Unfortunately, some of the squaddies who regarded sound once they boarded the troopships fell ill en direction and transmitted the flu to each one-of-a-kind.

A sailor on board couldn't manipulate his emotion as he watched the our bodies being buried at sea en masse. One day sooner or later of that experience from New York to France, 15 useless our our bodies were buried. The sailor recalled: "I confess I turn out to be close to to tears, and that there was tightening round my throat. It changed into loss of lifestyles, loss of life in one in every of its worst forms, to be consigned nameless to the sea."

Fighting the Spanish Flu Through Public Health Ordinances

Steps had been taken to reduce down or manage the spread of the sickness decrease decrease returned home whilst reality dawned on governments. Generally, officials imposed quarantines in some corporations. Movements were confined. Public locations which embody schools, church homes, theatres, consuming places, and department shops have been close down. All libraries brief stopped lending books. There have been suggestions and schooling on a way to cough or sneeze in public. Spitting in public emerge as absolutely prohibited.

People have been encouraged to stay at domestic and exit fine even as ultimately critical. Shaking of arms modified into to be avoided. At the height of it, there was lockdown. Violators of any of these regulations have been reminded or perhaps prosecuted thru mobile courts.

Public health officers allocated gauze nose mask for each person to place on if he had to go out. All shops, except food and shops, could not preserve profits. All wedding ceremony ceremonies had been positioned on keep. Funeral provider duration become constrained to fifteen minutes and attendance emerge as constrained handiest to the bereaved and the officiating ministers. Anyone who neglected the flu ordinances emerge as made to pay heavy fines.

In a few towns, passengers had to gift a signed certificates earlier than they is probably allowed to board train and railroads might no longer even accept all of us with out those certificates. Any transporter conveying uncertified passengers had violated the flu ordinances and should face the music.

Different Cities Different Initiatives in Fighting the Scourge

When the Spanish flu hit in 1918, scientists and a handful of scientific docs to be had could not affirm what caused it and a way to deal with it. Vaccine, no longer like in recent times, had no longer been evolved to enhance the frame's safety closer to microbes and antiviral have been truly non-existent. Hence, no drug changed into to be had to deal with flu sufferers.

The Center for Disease Control and Prevention became now not yet installed. The handiest component to do changed into to prevent man or woman-to-person transmission. This measure, they stated, might likely permit the virus to run its course inside the infected our our our bodies or kill the ones already inflamed. (The measure nevertheless works to date in the eradication of infectious sicknesses that defy treatments.)

To make certain this, life in lots of towns in the United States were added to a standstill in October 1918. Consider how unique cities spoke back to the scourge.

- San Francisco: Court intervals were held outdoor in public squares. Judges imposed discretionary fines on citizens who appeared in public with out sporting protecting gauze masks. The punishment for loss of "masks slackers" might also want to lure a few difficulty from $5 outstanding or to jail terms. Thus, you can see public posters ultimately of the cities with the inscription: "Obey the felony pointers, and placed on the gauze."

- New York City: This metropolis made a as a substitute uncommon selection. Instead of remaining the schools, the metropolis authority argued that youngsters is probably higher cared for while surrounded through faculty nurses than at the same time as staying at home inside the care of mother and father with very little understanding of stopping or treating the flu. Thus, the New York City Health Commissioner Royal Copeland decided to hold schools and specific public venues open. To bow to the mounting stress, Copeland directed staggered starting up and ultimate paintings hours for factories and corporations. This should decrease rush-hour crowds in those places and on subway trains.

- Philadelphia: One of the hardest-hit towns, Philadelphia's Public Health Director Wilmer Krusen first of all omitted medical doctors' pleas to cancel a parade wherein authorities struggle bonds had been to be promoted. He need to have stated higher. The event had 200,000 people in attendance, the bulk of whom went home with the Spanish flu virus. Commenting on this incident in his e book More Deadly Than War: The Hidden History of the Spanish Flu and the First World War, writer Kenneth C. Davis says: "Three days later each bed in the town's hospitals turned into crammed. Philadelphia become almost on the verge of ordinary fall apart as a functioning town."

Over 759 Philadelphians died on the worst day out of the outbreak in October. That very month, eleven,000 died in that city. It were given so lousy to the volume that drivers of open carts were continuously circling streets hollering, "Bring out your vain!" The town government excavated mass graves by using manner of way of steam shovel wherein piles of lifeless our our bodies have been given mass burial.

- Chicago: Even whilst human beings had been allowed to move, Chicago didn't relent in its attempt to sensitize masses. For instance, in public area posters and billboards have been visible with reminders and warnings. Playing their additives to gradual the spread of the flu, the control of one theater displayed a poster pronouncing: "Influenza often complicated with pneumonia is common proper now inside the path of America. This theater is co-operating with the branch of fitness. You have to do the identical. If you have got a cold and are coughing and sneezing, do no longer enter this theater. Go domestic and go to mattress till you're nicely. Help us to preserve Chicago the healthiest city within the global.—John Dill Robertson, Commissioner for Health."

A lot of various cities devised similar or a piece specific ingenuity to address the scourge. Red Cross, Boys Scout, and other voluntary corporations accomplished numerous roles in a unmarried-of-a-type cities to have the scourge in the end defeated.

Living in the Past?

One hundred years have exceeded due to the fact tens of loads of hundreds of mankind fell to the flu that ravaged America in a very massive way. But the scourge illustrates human beings' potential to heal emotional wounds. In spite of the lives misplaced, households bereaved, and lives changed for all time, the Spanish flu specially diminished brief from public reputation.

Nevertheless, it'll stay all the time in facts. Whenever the World War is remembered every November eleven, the havoc wreaked through the use of the Spanish flu that overlapped the conflict will hold to flash in the minds. Families may moreover additionally select out not to reflect onconsideration on all of it yet again because it become too horrible to assume. It need to be understood that this one of the strategies to deal with the flu whose imprints are however and will stay clean a long term to head back.

The U.S. Center for Disease Control and Prevention will take delivery of as real with historian Davis quoted earlier who gives: "The mixture of the flu and the conflict made Americans afraid of what changed into to be had within the wider global, so there has been a growing notion of becoming an isolationist u . S . And keeping out foreign elements. It combines for a period of tremendous fear—worry of communism, bolshevism and socialism."

Let's now shift the attention to how America overcame this scourge and music the improvement in stopping the disorder.

Chapter 7: Forever In America History

Looking at much less than four hundred citizens of non violent Brevig Mission in recent times from afar, you possibly can every now and then recollect how the village became wiped out some 100 years within the past. Before November 15, 1918, 80 adults had been living within the venture. But in the subsequent 5 days, 72 of them were killed before they may even understand their killer.

The contemporary-day residents of this assignment and places that suffered the equal fate will all the time have in records what the 1918 flu did to America and the manner it retarded the kingdom's development in the direction of restoration from the war. The story told as an example thru the 8 Brevig Mission survivors to the succeeding era will continue to be ever glowing of their minds.

How America Overcame It

Did America ever overcome the Spanish flu? Yes and no: it's miles predicated upon. Yes, Today's America is without a doubt free of Spanish flu and the sickness is nowhere to be decided now. Deliberate efforts to forestall the spread nationwide and internationally pay off. No, it wasn't eliminated thru only human intervention. Remember that there has been little expertise of the disorder. How come a person could declare that he treated the sufferers?

The virus atom definitely reduced and faded off at the identical time because it cannot be transmitted to every different character. The worldwide truely reached herd immunity; approximately fifty 5 percent is good enough to stifle the growth of the virus. But can it come decrease again? One hundred years is lengthy sufficient for the strain of the flu to move back lower again if it ever will. Spanish influenza will in no way go to the sector all once more!

Does that mean, however, that America can visit bed without making equipped for the following pandemic? No! That's why CDC has been away from bed for decades, caution within the path of the possibilities of a few other worldwide infectious contamination possibly lethal because the Spanish flu if now not managed.

Benefits of Hindsight

More than three pandemics have damaged out for the motive that 1918 pandemic. The years 1957, 1968, and 2009 each witnessed outbreaks of offspring of the HN viruses. Nevertheless, they had been a lot less excessive and their mortality fee changed into a whole lot less than the 1918 pandemic. Several unique viral outbreaks were controlled earlier than the could advantage their complete functionality of becoming each different worldwide pandemic. Scientists have tested the capability to lessen even the maximum present day day pandemic.

So does that endorse that the predictions of each distinct lethal and additional virulent virus attack can in no manner come right? It can besides the world sustains the continuing try to save you it. A particular virus unique that has garnered international hobby and has been a supply of situation is the avian influenza A (H7N9) virus from China. There are others too that, if allowed to unfold speedy and effectively among people, the pandemic they may motive will be extra intense than the Spanish flu pandemic.

A World Leveraging Vantage

While thinking about the opportunity of each other excessive severity pandemic in current instances, it's also critical to area it beside large scientific, scientific and societal achievements inside the international due to the truth 1918. Yes, there may be room for improvement, masses has been finished within the vicinity of vaccination and understanding of the homes of the virus.

Such subjects as scientific and diagnostic era and countermeasures had been virtually nonexistent in 1918. Doctors knew little or no longer something about viruses. There became not some thing like pandemic planning. Medical care, sickness surveillance and unique areas of fitness generation resulting in the production of the flu vaccine and antiviral tablets have been not to be had.

For instance, CDC in 2004 started out a 5-one year international surveillance ability constructing initiative that entailed monetary assist targeted at improving laboratory and diagnostic checks. It additionally adds surveillance of influenza-like ailments.

With initiatives which incorporates the ones, it's far obvious that even though the pandemic moves, the U.S. Will conquer it earlier than it receives out of hand.

Spanish Flu Timeline

What happened earlier than, throughout, and right away after the flu as contained in this timeline will function further proof that America can beat any pandemic.

Date Event

March eleven, 1918 Influenza-like signs and symptoms are counseled early inside the morning with the useful resource of an Army Private at Fort Riley. Over 100 soldiers have similar signs and symptoms and 48 infantrymen died at Fort Riley.

May 1918 Public health officials in Philadelphia warn approximately what they nicknamed "Spanish influenza" after Spain begins reporting it.

September 1918 Dr. Victor Vaughn visits Camp Devens close to Boston and sees pretty a few unwell more youthful guys manifesting first-rate flu signs and symptoms and symptoms and symptoms. Sixty 3 of them die of influenza that day. A lot of scientific quackery isn't any healthy for the ravaging sickness. It proves to be simply trial and mistakes.

September five, 1918 The Massachusetts Department of Health tells the neighborhood press that they'll be preventing a virus. According to one of the docs with the Massachusetts State Health Department, "until precautions are taken the infection in all probability will unfold to the civilian populace of the city."

September 13, 1918

Rupert Blue, the Surgeon General inside the United States Public Health Service issued a press launch on spotting the influenza signs and symptoms and signs and signs in order to proscribing its unfold. He prescribes bed rest, real hygiene, an excellent weight-reduction plan, and aspirin for the sick. But the Health Commissioner of New York City, Royal Copeland, proclaims, "The town is in no risk of a deadly disease. No want for our humans to fear."

September 24, 1918 The San Francisco public fitness officials who have downplayed the risk of the flu, giving fake assurances to the overall public are in wonder even as Edward Wagner, newly transplanted from Chicago, catches the flu.

September 28, 1918

America has a desire to make among shutting the whole lot all the way all of the manner right down to lessen the spread of influenza and speeding the whole thing as an awful lot as win the war. A incorrect preference is made and the sickness spreads.

Philadelphia moreover involves a decision to maintain a large earnings parade. The quit quit result is disastrous.

Congress approves $1 million to research into the flu and paintings on a vaccine.

October 2, 1918

The loss of lifestyles toll in Boston reaches 202. The Liberty Bond parades, in addition to all wearing activities, are canceled. The inventory market additionally begins offevolved half of-day operations.

October three, 1918

Influenza reaches Seattle, Washington. Seven-hundred times are recorded with surely one death. They are taken to the University of Washington Naval Training Station.

October 6, 1918   The day Philadelphia statistics 289 influenza-associated deaths.

October 7, 1918   New Mexico, which had managed to be flu-free up till now evaluations its first case.

October 11, 1918   Santa Fe in New Mexico reviews its first flu-associated demise.

October 15, 1918   851 New Yorkers die in a unmarried day. Meanwhile, the crime charge in Chicago drops thru forty 3 percent.

October 19, 1918 Dr. C.Y. White announces in Philadelphia that he has superior a vaccine which could prevent the Spanish flu. More than 10,000 series of inoculations are sent to the Philadelphia Board of Health for approval. Under the auspices of the USA Public Health Services, researchers art work on vaccines however they get all of it wrong as they may be targeted on the bacterium. No outcomes are visible among hundreds of humans inoculated.

October 29, 1918 Seattle authorities mandate using six-ply gauze masks.

October 30, 1918 The use of six-ply gauze masks becomes compulsory within the whole united states of america of Washington.

October 31, 1918 Most Halloween celebrations are canceled due to the

Influenza pandemic that is ravaging national.

The influenza mortality charge reaches 195,000 in America all through October.

Armed guards are employed through funeral houses to prevent the ones stealing coffins.

November 1, 1918 Because a few human beings refuse to vicinity on the mask, violence erupts and people are being shot. There are homicides and suicides as people finish that their households, loved ones, and pals, will inflict them.

November three, 1918 New precautions closer to the flu are launched. Masses are advised to easy in the nostril with cleansing soap and water each morning and night; spark off sneeze morning and night time time time; exercising deep respiration; refrain from wearing a muffler; take brisk walks often; trek back home from paintings; and eat plenty of porridge.

November eleven, 1918 World War 1 ends! Armistice is delivered! People troop out with celebration forgetting the continued pandemic. Everyone is unfastened to transport about in the street in all elements of the arena. They are out with out their masks, having been carried away through manner of the Armistice. Unfortunately, that leads to huge infection with flu and this results in a surge in influenza instances.

November 18, 1918 By this date, five,000 New Mexicans have died.

November 21, 1918 An declaration is going spherical in sirens sound in San Francisco that everybody is free to move about with out face mask.

December 1918 San Francisco reviews some exceptional five,000 instances of influenza.

January 1919 All faculties reopen in Seattle.

March 1919 Zero influenza deaths are said in Seattle.

The timeline can keep till the existing second.

Chapter 8: Virus' Analysis

In 1918, a pressure of flu called Spanish influenza brought about a worldwide pandemic, spreading speedy and killing indiscriminately. Youthful, antique, debilitated, and in any other case healthful human beings all got infected, and at any charge, 10% of sufferers died.

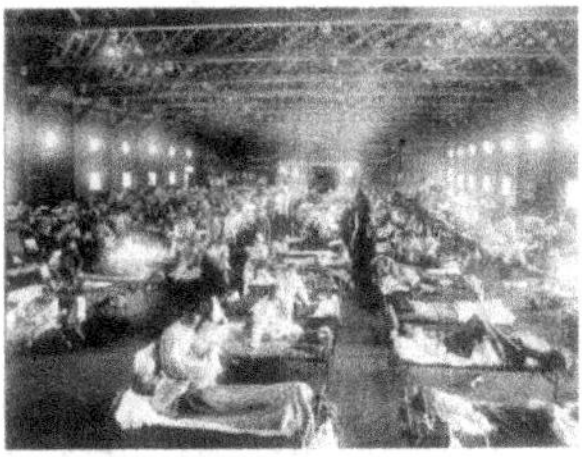

2 - Emergency navy hospital[2]

Estimates range at the correct quantity of deaths introduced about with the useful aid of the illness. However, it's far perception to have infected 33% of the complete population and killed in any occasion 50 million humans, making it the deadliest pandemic in current-day information. Although on the time it picked up the nickname "Spanish flu," it's far now not going that the virus started in Spain.

WHAT CAUSED SPANISH INFLUENZA?

The outbreak started in 1918, over the past period of a completely long time of World War I, and historians currently take transport of that the struggle may additionally were without a doubt chargeable for spreading the virus. On the Western Front, officers living in cramped, grimy, and damp situations have become out to be sick. This emerge as a direct end stop end result of debilitated safe frameworks from malnourishment. Their diseases, that have been called "I. A.

Grippe," have been infectious, and unfold maximum of the positions. Around three days of getting unwell, numerous warriors must begin to feel suitable, but no longer all could probable make it.

Throughout the mid-12 months of 1918, as troops started out to move once more home on depart, they carried with them the hidden contamination that had made them sick. The virus unfold at some stage in town areas, cities, and villages inside the squaddies' domestic countries. A huge range of these inflamed, soldiers and civilians, failed to recover fast. The infection modified into hardest on extra youthful adults between the a long term of 20 and 30 who had these days been healthful.

In 2014, every other hypothesis about the birthplaces of the virus endorsed that it formerly superior in China, National Geographic stated. Previously undiscovered facts related this season's cold virus to the transportation of Chinese human beings, the Chinese Labor Corps, within the path of Canada in 1917 and 1918. The personnel were, for the maximum issue, farmworkers from the a long way off elements of China, as indicated through way of Mark Humphries' ebook, "The Last Plague" (University of Toronto Press, 2013). They went through six days in consistent educate containers as they have been transported throughout the united states of the united states over earlier than intending to France. There, they had been required to burrow channels, empty trains, lay tracks, manufacture streets, and join harmed tanks. Taking all matters collectively, extra than ninety,000 clinical docs had been prepared in the direction of the Western Front.

Humphries clarifies that out of 25,000 Chinese human beings in 1918, almost three,000 completed their Canadian adventure in scientific quarantine. At that component, and in moderate of racial stereotypes, their disease come to be blamed on "Chinese laziness," and Canadian professionals did not be aware of the people' signs and symptoms. When the human beings confirmed up in northern France in mid-1918, many have been unwell, and loads have been quick demise.

FOR WHAT REASON WAS IT CALLED THE SPANISH FLU?

Spain became perhaps the earliest america in which the plague grow to be identified. However, information experts receive this emerge as in all likelihood a end result of wartime censorship. Spain become an impartial u . S . A . During the conflict and did now not uphold extreme control of its press, which could therefore freely put up early debts of the contamination. Subsequently, human beings falsely well-known the disease became particular to Spain, and the decision "Spanish flu" stuck.

Indeed, even in past due spring 1918, a Spanish records issuer reached out to

Reuters' London place of work advising the statistics employer that "an amazing form of infection of epidemic man or woman has shown up in Madrid. The plague is of a mellow type, no passing having been accounted for," Inside about fourteen days of the file, more than 100,000 people had gotten infected with the flu.

The infection struck the lord of Spain, Alfonso XIII, along main politicians. Anywhere in the sort of 30% and forty% of those who worked or lived in restrained areas, for example, colleges, army quarters, and authorities houses, have become infected. Administration on the Madrid cable vehicle framework need to be reduced, and the telegraph company become disturbed within the instances due to the fact there have been no longer sufficient healthy personnel to be had to paintings. Clinical components and offerings couldn't stay aware about the hobby.

The expression "Spanish flu" fast grabbed maintain in Britain. As indicated through the usage of Niall Johnson's e-book "England and the 1918-19 Influenza Pandemic" (Routledge, 2006), the British press accused this season's flu virus plague in Spain for the Spanish climate: "... the dry, breezy Spanish spring is an scary and terrible season," check one article in The Times. It have become proposed that microbe-laden dirt become being unfold by using the excessive breezes in Spain, implying that Britain's moist climate also can stop the flu from spreading there.

WHAT WERE THE SYMPTOMS OF THE FLU?

Initial signs and symptoms and signs of the infection incorporated an angry head and tiredness, trailed by using way of way of a dry, hacking cough; misplaced yearning; belly problems; and then, on a next day, extreme perspiring. Next, the disorder also can want to affect the respiration organs, and pneumonia must expand. Humphries clarifies that pneumonia, or exceptional respiratory problems completed through the usage of this flu, have been often the principle motives of dying. This clarifies why it is tough to determine specific numbers killed through the flu, due to the reality the recorded purpose for demise become often some thing apart from the flu.

By mid-twelve months of 1918, the contamination changed into unexpectedly spreading to special global locations inside the terrain of Europe. Vienna, Budapest and Hungary had been enduring, and components of Germany and France have been additionally brought on. Numerous youngsters in Berlin colleges were accounted for as unwell and lacking from college, and absences in armament factories decreased production.

By June 25, 1918, this flu epidemic in Spain had arrived at the British. In July, the epidemic modified into putting the London fabric change tough, with one production plant having 80 out of 4 hundred medical doctors go lower back domestic wiped out in one night by myself. In London, it covers authorities employees lacking due to the reality seasonal influenza is going from 25% to 1/2 of of the employees.

The epidemic had rapid gotten to a virulent disease, advancing a protracted manner and big. Around the identical time, instances have been accounted for some of the Swedish armed stress, at that aspect within the u.S.'s civilian populace, and among South Africa's going for walks population. By September, this flu had arrived on the U.S. Through Boston harbor.

DEVELOPMENT

At the hour of the 1918 pandemic, clinical professionals did now not have any idea approximately its causes, and closer to the start, there were no effective remedies. Before the quit of the pandemic, treatment through the use of transfusion of blood from a survivor turn out to be stated to be compelling. However, transfusion techniques have been simple, completed without delay from benefactor to affected person, and blood typing and matching were in its beginning.

3 - Nurse carrying a masks as safety in opposition to influenza. September 13, 1918[3]

Researchers felt that flu modified into brought about with the aid of manner of the usage of a bacterium they known as Baccilus influenzae (presently referred to as Hemophilus influenzae.) They can also additionally need to isolate and phrase severa forms of bacteria underneath a microscope. They moreover realized that there have been contamination professionals littler than microbes that they will sieve through a mixture. Not having the option to look the ones rather little professionals, there has been a talk about whether they had been chemical substances or quite small organisms. However, vaccines in opposition to those extremely small dealers, which they known as viruses, had just been created returning to the smallpox vaccine within the overdue 18th century.

In the a long time following the pandemic, researchers remembered the hazard of flu and attempted to build up a advanced comprehension of the sickness. In 1931, Richard Shope taken into consideration pigs conveying pig influenza, and accomplished strategies applied earlier than some years to end up aware about the motives for yellow fever and wonderful ailments. He located that the presence of H. Flu made swine flu worse, however did not purpose it. In 1936, Shope indicated that human beings living and coping with the pig farms had antibodies to pig influenza, demonstrating that the human and swine sickness had been firmly associated. Contemporary scientists created strategies to view such little particles using electron microscopes, and chemically distinguished them as being made up essentially of protein and ribonucleic acids.

In 1931, an big development end up made at Vanderbilt University. Analysts there placed approaches to extend the flu virus in rich chook eggs. This supposed they not had to get them from unwell people or animals. Growing viruses and searching at immunological reactions of lab animals, scientists recognized styles of flu infections, referred to as them A and B. The 1918 pandemic contamination become a Type A infection. Today we understand that Type A infections infect each people and some distinct animals and are more dangerous. Type B infections are in people simplest.

With the potential to boom quantities of the viruses, and to choose out their functions, analysts inside the late Nineteen Thirties started out jogging on a vaccine. In 1937, with stress to get equipped for a few distinctive battle developing, British analysts tried a vaccine on officers, and in 1938 america Army started out out out an ordeal of vaccines with an exploration organization that covered Jonas Salk. The first mass utilization of flu vaccines for officers in the United States came in 1944, and for everyday humans, in 1945. During the exploration of this immunization, it have end up determined that invulnerability towards one shape of contamination would now not provide immunity in opposition to the opposite. So the vaccine contained a combination of the two kinds and a trouble of reference no matter everything determined in recent times.

The exploration of the virus, and inoculation to save you the flu, delivered approximately numerous disclosures. It made equipment for the development of numerous vaccines. Today we, despite everything, make use of ripe eggs to boom infections. It moreover caused our thoughts on the idea of capabilities and the chemicals that encode them. Oswald Avery, an analyst on the Rockefeller Institute, led the organization that determined in 1944 that deoxyribonucleic acid (DNA) held the genetic code. Their studies carried out machine created in recognizing the additives and varieties of viruses and used a micro organism that motives pneumonia. Avery's work turn out to be based mostly on the huge artwork of Frederick Griffith's art work that Avery at the start got down to disprove. Unfortunately, Griffiths, who modified right into a British researcher, died within the Blitz in 1941.

Although there had been attempts at vaccination at some point of the pandemic, the useful version of flu vaccines in the United States commenced sooner or later of the 1940s. Thomas Francis Jr. And Jonas Salk, higher seemed later for their art work on the polio antibody, were instrumental within the improvement of influenza immunizations. The maximum crucial permitted version of the immunization have grow to be controlled to squaddies in 1945, for the duration of World War II. Regular parents had the choice to get vaccinated the following year.

Flu viruses can transform thru antigenic go with the flow and shift, which calls for commonly adapting vaccine types. Since adopting new measures in 1973, the World Health Organization (WHO) includes a choice the 3, absolute confidence flu traces or candidate vaccine viruses (CVVs), to take into account for that three hundred and sixty five days's influenza shot. There are likewise quadrivalent immunizations to be had.

Up to this point, nearly all flu vaccines have been fabricated utilising prepared chicken eggs to propagate the virus. This technique includes turning into every one of the 3 anticipated CVVs in separate eggs and becoming a member of the 3 into one vaccine. One of the essential factors of hobby to this technique is that eggs are a lot much less steeply-priced and unfold flu to excessive titers. There are dangers, however. In some unusual examples, the egg-based completely completely vaccines have introduced approximately allergic reactions. If an avian flu strain had been to get unstable, it may weigh down bird populations and cause a lack of eggs for utilization or vaccine production, which befell in 2015 with the exceedingly pathogenic H5N2. There are currently viral vectored vaccines available now which could help the fowl makers if every other H5 episode like this takes place; those inoculations uses Charles River's Specific Pathogen Free (SPF) cells or eggs.

In any case, egg-primarily based methods can be tedious and flighty, with a multi-month slack among CVV segregation and completed immunizations, and adjustments in the degree of immunization accumulated from every egg. In this way, flu vaccine producers are searching out alternatives.

Then once more, experts had been chipping away at cellular-based totally completely vaccines to replace the identical old egg approach. In 2016, the U.S. Food and Drug Administration (FDA) popular the manufacturing of Novartis' antibody Flucelvax utilising cell-primarily based completely virus isolation. In this method, cultured animal cells are implemented to incubate the viruses in preference to eggs. This approach no longer simply eliminates the ability problem of an influenza outbreak, but additionally lets in for faster assembling; but, it is not quicker than conventional techniques wherein flu in eggs incubates in 48-seventy two hours.

Since the Spanish influenza emergency, there have been three more flu pandemics, maximum as of past due in 2009. Luckily, due to the fact the discovery of vaccines and one-of-a-type advances in modern-day-day social coverage, none have been about as savage because the 1918 pandemic. In any case, without a normal flu vaccine and with fantastic humans not worthy or reluctant to get a every 12 months shot, it is just a short time earlier than some different outbreak takes place. Flu is a doubtful contamination and has even stood out as in reality newsworthy this one year, with new lines being placed in dogs. In any case, with always advancing technology like cell-based vaccines, destiny docs are organized to installation a combat in competition to the flu.

Chapter 9: Origins And Causes

THREE WAVES OF SPANISH FLU

First Wave: Springtime in Spain, 1918

Sache stayed unbiased throughout World War I. As the end of the conflict drew closer in 1918, the u . S . Faced a complex public and political situation. Alfonso XIII, the King of Spain, managed a socially divided u.S. With the huge majority of its close to 20,000,000 residents ruined, given the lack of trade and resources that came about thinking about that the beginning of World War I. In Spain, the swelling price have become the most (20.1%) it have been due to the truth the start of the twentieth century. There end up an growing price of social elegance clashes, together with a few great moves.

The first public information of the epidemic confirmed up in Madrid. On 22 May 1918, the flu scourge become a name text in Madrid's ABC paper. News expressed that the unfold of a peculiar influenza-like contamination, that have grow to be pretty moderate, have been non-stop because the begin of May. Due to Madrid's every year close by vacations (Fiesta de San Isidro), an remarkable style of people assembled in meeting halls and famous gatherings (Verbenas) at a few stage inside the zero.33 seven day stretch of May and, in this way, have been probable furnished to a immoderate risk of virus transmission. The said contamination grow to be a surprising one; some people actually have fallen whilst strolling on the road. The disease delivered as a 2–three-day fever, gastrointestinal thing effects, and present day tension and became associated with a totally low dying fee. After seven days (28 May), King Alfonso XIII have become out to be sick, as did the Prime Minister and a few cabinet individuals. Many humans remained at home from paintings given the sickness, and a few simple offerings, which encompass the postal and telegraph offerings, and some banks and saving debts offices needed to in brief close operations. The plague modified into every day information round then, underneath the function "La Epidemia refinance" ("The Prevailing Epidemic"). As a give up quit result of the perceived loss of severity of the ailment and due to Spanish comical inclination, the flu modified into stated prominently in Madrid due to the fact the "Soldado de Napoles" ("Naples Soldier"), that have end up the decision of a mainstream melody from an incredibly fruitful melodic, La canción Del Olvido, which have become gambling concurrently at Madrid's Teatro de los angeles Zarzuela. The song modified into widely recognized to such an amount that it become deemed to be "relatively contagious," like flu.

A few observers recommended that the pestilence might have been spread from France because of the overwhelming railroad website visitors of unskilled Spanish and Portuguese professionals to and from

France, who gave transitory substitution to the dearth of more youthful French humans engaged in the struggle. Besides a historic competition amongst France and Spain, this is the possibly reason why, in Spain, the flu have emerge as in any other case known as the French flu. As a stop end result in their ordinary journey through manner of railroad, the ones migrant humans were a feasible hotspot for the advent and spread of the flu infection in Spain. Beginning in focal and southern France (near the battlefields and Army camps) and following the railway manner path from north to east (Portugal), and from north to south (Andalusia), the flu unfold sooner or later of just about everything of Spain's regions. Death fees related to flu in this first time of the pandemic prolonged from zero.04 to 0.Sixty 5 deaths in step with one thousand population. The fashionable loss of life price multiplied exceptional barely in a few unspecified time in the future of this number one plague period. The unknown and elusive etiology of the pandemic in addition hampered and discredited the paintings of public fitness physicians, who've been examined every day through the press. However, the primary period of the epidemic was over all of sudden. About 2 months after the reality, the whole thing seemed to have again to normal.

Second Wave: Autumn and wintry climate in Spain, 1918

The second time of the pandemic showed up progressively in severa factors of Spain in September 1918, arriving at its top in October and waning in December 1918.

It is difficult to verify whether or now not the A (H1N1) virus was reintroduced to Spain from France or whether or now not the virus changed into all of the on the identical time as circling inside the united states. General fitness authorities acknowledged the giant process that the railway transportation system might also play in the unfold of the epidemic. Several infection-control measures in vital inland educate stations and middle factors have been carried out. Trains stacked with Portuguese specialists were halted in Spain, halfway to Portugal, and tourists were no longer allowed to depart the educate until it left over again to Portugal. Spanish navy making equipped camps went approximately as an inexperienced diffusion device; ill navy personnel with flu have been relieved from duty and sent home thru train to rest and get hospital treatment.

When the influenza virus took place in a Spanish city or metropolis, most in all likelihood carried there via way of migrant human beings or through military college, there was every other trouble that endorsed its spread. Toward the surrender of the mid-one year, a huge form of Spanish cities celebrated their conventional holidays with well-known sports and profoundly went to Catholic Mass festivals. In high-quality times, flu turn out to be even wrong for foodborne illness, due to the truth about the whole lot of the people going to those activities have emerge as out to be ill some days later.

Influenza-related mortality quotes had been very immoderate, extending from 0.5 to fourteen.Zero deaths in keeping with 1000 inhabitants. The imply month to month massive sort of deaths of all reasons become decided for the duration 1913–1917 and modified into plotted in competition to the watched variety of passings for the length September-December 1918. This rely gave the greater big style of deaths at some level in the second one time of the influenza epidemic.

The common lifestyles of Spaniards changed into disturbed. School and college phrases had been canceled, but specific public gatherings, for example, the ones at church services or theaters and movies, proceeded. There were difficult stressful situations whilst seeking out to execute public health-manipulate measures. Public health officials in Valladolid, Spain, argued with neighborhood authorities approximately officially putting forward that there was a progressing plague due to the fact that close by holidays (and the related commercial enterprise company) were at their pinnacle. The contention that at closing persuaded the authorities covered the compensation framework for human provider workers. If a physician died of the contamination at the equal time as on the interest and if there was now not yet a plague scenario formally declared, at that detail, the widow have emerge as no longer certified for getting a finance enjoy the government. Doctors placed the overwhelming attention on the civic chairman of Valladolid, and the flu pandemic turned into consequently formally announced in Spain.

The city Zamora had one of the most extended loss of lifestyles charges in Spain, arriving at a top of 10.1% in October 1918 (with the aid of and massive flu loss of life price in Spain around the equal time become 3.8%). It ranked 2nd to Burgos (flu-associated death charge in October 1918 modified into 12.1%). As a forestall end result of a robust social impact of the Bishop, the Catholic Church experts in Zamora expressed that "the evil upon us may be an very last consequences of our sins and lack of gratitude, and this manner the vengeance of eternal justice felt upon us," and as a end result, organized a development of Mass social sports at Zamora's Cathedral. One of the possibly effects of the sports have grow to be the smooth unfold of the contamination. The efforts of civil authorities to forbid Mass get-togethers have been puzzled thru the Bishop, who blamed the govt and public fitness establishments of excessive obstruction with the church. Every day Mass proceeded with appreciably huge audiences in a tough scenario and misery. A everyday supplication spherical then have come to be an vintage one named Pro tempore pestilentia (For the Times of Pestilence), which asked God that people be stored from plague and starvation, and communicated the humans' conviction that it come to be God's will that they had been pressured and that God's kindness should cease the tribulation.

Public fitness movements acquired with the resource of political professionals protected cleansing with phenolic oil or creoline (Zotal, a well-known disinfectant at that thing). The Spanish Royal Academy of Medicine requested the muse and the viability of those techniques; but, the assessment of community authorities prevailed, and tourists, their matters, and railroad and tramway wagons were purified. Theaters, cafeterias, and church homes have been furthermore disinfected. Indeed, even the mail modified into wiped clean. In a few Spanish metropolis areas, avenues were wiped easy with a mixture of water and sodium hypochlorite, and spitting became confined. In Madrid, the Congress and the Senate systems had been also disinfected.

Doctors and Public Health Officials encouraged some measures to save you influenza transmission. These measures blanketed cleaning and sanitizing the mouth and nostrils with hydrogen peroxide or a combination of oil and menthol, staying away from gatherings or social sports in closed settings, avoiding direct touch with sick people, ingesting a wholesome weight-reduction plan, frequently strolling in new outside, ventilating homes, and periodic resting. These simple measures had been frequently tough to look at, especially for the lowest-profits populace.

The Spanish Health System changed into overpowered and failed to deliver a effective response. Numerous little towns unfold across america of a desired clinical help; their medical clinical docs died, and the substitute changed into difficult (some volunteer scientific college college students have been deployed).

The little show off of medication recommended included indicative remedy with salicylates and quinine and codeine for cough. For folks who created pneumonia, the remedial alternatives have been drastically a whole lot much less and blanketed intramuscular or intravenous remedy with silver or platinum colloid arrangements, digitalis, alcamphoroil, or adrenaline. Draining become frequently applied. Some trial vaccines have been moreover attempted, drastically those at the side of combinations of pneumococci, streptococci, and Pfeiffer bacillus (Haemophilus influenzae). All efforts come to be being nearly futile, and Spaniards started thinking about all yet again whether or not or not clinical experts and researchers had any idea of what changed into occurring.

In light of the excessive demise charge, burial service homes and houses of church homes have been besieged. Some Spanish town areas ran out of coffins. The chairman of Barcelona cited the military's help for the transportation and burial of the vain because town corridor people at the manner had been scared. Some tremendous prison recommendations were showed, which includes the suspension of the equal antique 2–3-day memorial carrier capabilities that drove towards the Dead Mass (Corpore insepulto), which closes with the internment of the frame as consistent with the Catholic rites. Corpses had been ordered to be buried as fast as time lets in, with out the same old prolonged services. Indeed, even the normal church ringer's fee for the lifeless from the 16th century (Toque de difuntos), defined by means of manner of its rushing up, and have become constrained in sure cities to keep away from further panic and demoralization of the populace. The Spanish papers of that factor commonly dedicated the primary web web page or pages to obituaries; in some unspecified time inside the future of the height of the second scourge time frame, upwards of four or five pages were carried out for obituaries.

Third Wave: Winter and spring in Spain, 1919

The 1/3 and very last time of the influenza epidemic in Spain occurred from January thru June 1919. The seriousness and period of this period have been milder than the ones of the previous pandemic time frame. It essentially motivated the regions of Spain in which the fundamental scourge came about, and it stored maximum of the regions that were generally precipitated continuously. Death costs went from 0.07 to at the least one.Forty deaths regular with a thousand occupants. The favored quantity of folks that died on of flu in Spain were authoritatively assessed to be 147,114 in 1918, 21,235 in 1919, and 17,825 in 1920.

If the commonplace epidemiological index for deaths because of pneumonia and flu is implemented, in moderate of professional morbidity and mortality figures, nearly actually more than 260,000 Spaniards died; nearly seventy five% of these humans died at a few level within the second time of the pestilence, and 45% died in October 1918. The mortality format related to the Spanish flu that became visible some different area have become additionally located in Spain; lack of existence prices had been better amongst people elderly a first rate deal much less than1 yr and amongst the ones elderly 25–29 years.

In vast, the loss of existence rate in 1918 turned into the maximum noteworthy in Spain in the twentieth century. The population growth (net increase of populace) have become poor in Spain simply instances sooner or later of the 20th century: in 1918 (identified with the flu pandemic; internet benefit, −83.121 people) and in 1939 (identified with the Spanish Civil War; net gain, −50.266 people). The extra mortality related to the 1918–1920 flu pandemic in Spain changed into 1.Forty 9% (90 5% CI, 1.Forty seven%–1.50%).

A few evaluations advocated that more than 8 million Spaniards advanced flu, yet a few Spanish authors left out this determine as overvalued. In 1918, a Medical Journal from British advocated about this discern: "The flu that we look at a good buy approximately inside the everyday papers appears to had been especially far-achieving in Spain within the route of the extended stretch of May; that there have been eight million instances of the contamination in that state, because the French press claimed at that point, is a statement requiring probably a grain of salt for deglutition; however, it in reality highlighted a substantial price". Considering the posted price within the 1918–1919 Spanish influenza pandemic, it isn't always unexpected that a excessive huge fashion of human beings obtained the infection; however, most expert a gentle and more not unusual medical presentation. The lack of incredibly solid morbidity information blocks any moreover subtle investigation of this statistics.

A couple of months after its starting, the presence of the plague emerge as identified outside Spain: "Flu exists glaringly in each u.S. Of the us in Europe, and in North, West, and South Africa; in India, in addition to in the North American Continent. The commonness pestilence this yr occurred first in Spain in May. The Canadian Medical Association Journal said that,, "Under the choice of Spanish flu, an epidemic is sweeping over the North American Continent. It is said to have showed up first in Spain, ultimately referred to as Spanish flu".

The 1918–1919flu pandemic grow to be the worst pandemic that has occurred in Spain. It placed extraordinary weight on the overall public health and medical structures and medical professionals. The pandemic became maximum likely chargeable for over 260,000 deaths (1% of the Spanish populace), with more mortality of near 1.Five%.

The flu pandemic changed into stated international because of the reality the Spanish flu. Since the pandemic, Spain has been added to a verifiable short rundown of nations with contamination-related names. Albeit a few global places are currently claiming Spanish flu as their very non-public and virologists and disease transmission specialists agree that the infection maximum likely did no longer begin in Spain, however the 1918 flu pandemic will generally be called the Spanish influenza pandemic. Spain and the remainder of the arena should constantly do not forget the caution that have become acquired.

This flu that converted the arena

Pathologist Jeffery Taubenberger of america National Institute of Allergy and Infectious Diseases – the individual that's 2005, together along with his partner Ann Reid, posted the genetic collection of the virus responsible for the pandemic, stated at an ongoing conference that there had been as however severa unanswered fantastic questions.

Analysts everywhere at a few diploma inside the international are strolling to reply them. Yet, what they've got absolutely revealed might also moreover marvel you.

The fittest were some of the maximum prone

Austrian craftsman Egon Schiele died of flu in October 1918, handiest multiple days after his large different Edith, who have become pregnant with their first toddler, died. Then, desperately sick and grieving, he took a shot at a painting that depicted a family of his very own that might in no manner exist.

Schiele changed into 28 years of age, solidly indoors an age organisation that established immoderate helplessness in competition to the 1918 influenza. It is one motivation behind why his unfinished portray, The Family, is frequently depicted as a poignant testimony to the contamination's cruelty.

Since it turned into so volatile to 20-to-forty-twelve months-olds, the sickness robbed families in their companies and businesses in their columns, leaving massive portions of vintage human beings and orphans with none approach of help. Men were usually at excessive chance of demise, in evaluation to the girls, besides for the women that have been pregnant, wherein scenario, they died or suffered miscarriages in droves.

Researchers do not know precisely why the ones in the excessive of existence have been so inclined. However, a probable explanation is the fact that the older people, instead of being at a excessive-danger of lack of lifestyles of influenza, were in fact, an entire lot less likely to die within the 1918 pandemic due to the reality they had been in influenza seasons during the earlier decade.

One speculation that in all likelihood clarifies each observations is "specific antigenic sin," – the possibility that a person's immune tool develops its splendid reaction to the number one pressure of influenza it studies. Influenza is a specially labile infection, implying that it changes its shape continuously but remembering that of the 2 primary antigens for its ground, diagnosed through the shorthand H and N, that attract with the host's immune tool.

As in line with the National Archives, "One-5th of the sector's population changed into attacked with the useful resource of this bad virus. Within months, it had killed a larger variety of human beings than some extraordinary ailments in written statistics. This flu greater than 25 percentage of the U.S. Populace. In 3 hundred and sixty 5 days, the everyday life expectancy within the United States dropped through 12 years."

For social and financial experts, the 1918 influenza pandemic and the surrender of World War 1 marked the begin of a complicated set of social, political, and economic sports that preserve on affecting up until these days.

Locally, 1918 marked the quit of the "Brilliant Age" of horticulture. Before 1918, the ranch have become the social, monetary, and political attention in Carroll County.

After World War I, that center moved to the numerous number one avenues of Carroll County's numerous humble communities. At approximately a comparable time, Westminster turned into looking ahead to the project of the focal point of an undeniably bureaucratized district authorities. It have become turning into an green social, monetary, and exchange attention.

For severa historians, the duration is stated because the "Lost Generation." The time period changed into first begat via Gertrude Stein, who were given the idea from her vehicle expert. From 1914 via 1918, round one hundred million of the human beings conceived someplace inside the range of 1883 and 1900 handed on from World War I or the flu.

One of the quick results of the "Lost Generation" on society come to be the way of women within the public eye have grow to be typically modified as they left the farms and entered the industrial and mechanical employees in unparalleled numbers.

As an outcome of the loss or absence of such massive numbers of fellows, girls started out to count on management roles. They have emerge as an financial stress that asked funding in selecting community options. This dynamic accelerated ladies being given the selection to solid a ballot thru the nineteenth Amendment in 1920.

The expression "the misplaced age" has been applied to awesome agencies of people who were alive within the mid-twentieth century, together with the talented American artists who got here of age eventually of the First World War and the British defense pressure officers whose lives have been stopped by way of that conflict.

In any case, it could pretty be argued, as I do in my e-book Pale Rider, that the credit score have to go to a super many human beings within the crucial of lifespan who surpassed away of the 1918 flu, or to the children who've been stranded through it, or to those, now not however conceived, who continued its slings and bolts in their moms' bellies.

The idea of the 1918 pandemic, and of logical statistics at that point, manner that we don't know exactly how many people were inside the ones three organizations; but, we can be fine that they includeeveryone dwarfed each the Jazz-Age artists and the 35,000-weird British officials who died in combat (South Africa had an expected 500,000 "flu orphans" on my own).

The folks who survived this flu virus in utero in idea lived with the scars till they died. Research indicates that they've been a whole lot less inclined to graduate or earn an inexpensive revenue, and are certain to visit jail, than pals who hadn't been inflamed.

What range of human beings died from Spanish flu?

Exactly 100 years in advance, 33% of the arena's population observed itself infected in a lethal viral pandemic. It come to be Spanish influenza. Its lack of life is unknown; but, considered to be greater than 50 million for the maximum component.

Some researchers have expected a loss of life fee as excessive as 10 to 20%.

During World War I in Europe, influenza struck squaddies and regular citizens inside the spring of 1918, and it erupted later within the U.S., in which 675,000 individuals passed away.

In the autumn of that twelve months, a in addition rush of the contamination crushed the globe, Bristow said. The younger and the vintage had been hard hit, but middle-aged, and anyways, sound people moreover suffered; those aged 20-40 represented approximately the part of the deaths within the pandemic.

"What's noteworthy is this have come to be infectious enough that it appears to have arrived in locations for which there may be no apparent touch," Bristow said, referring to an Inuit town in Alaska, where seventy two out of eighty populace bypass away from the 1918 flu inside the span of five days.

Around 50 to 100 million people have been killed spherical the world, as indicated through Amesh Adalja, an infectious disease health practitioner and senior investigator on the Johns Hopkins Center for Health Security. He places the passing charge from the 1918 pestilence at spherical 1 to 2% globally.

Different teachers have assessed the demise price from the pandemic to run from 10 to twenty%.

All the numbers are first rate estimates. "In 1918, passing testament recording, and the take a look at of disorder transmission became honestly in its earliest degrees," stated Adalja. "We did not have the whole lot of that information. What's extra, numerous components of the area were now not related to particular parts of the sector. So you couldn't get facts from part of the bad asset zones that existed round then."

Bristow, Adalja, and unique teachers generally agree that this season's bloodless virus pandemic sickened round 500 million people.

As a bargain as the drugs is stopping with the present infection, clinical doctors had even a splendid deal an awful lot much less to venture with a century lower back.

"The 1918 pandemic changed into the maximum excessive pandemic that we have were given on report," stated Adalja. "We had no ICUs round then. We had no vaccines, had no inoculations for flu. We had no clue that this season's bloodless virus changed into even a virus round then."

One hassle is for exquisite, and the 1918 pandemic proved that social preserving aside is strong, as in line with Bristow.

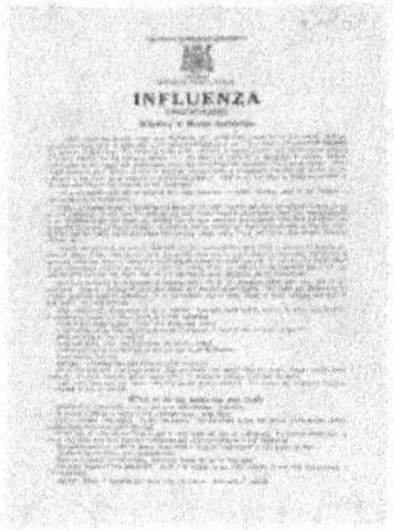
INFLUENZA

four - Influenza Poster[4]

Chapter 10: Consequences Of Virus

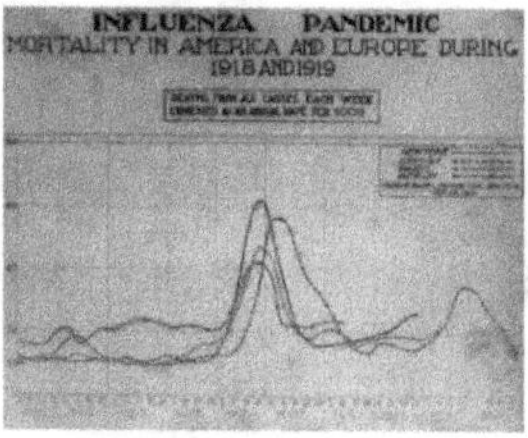

SPANISH INFLUENZA ORPHANS

5 - Chart of Mortality[5]

Fowl it reduced in 1920, Spanish influenza had killed 675,000 Americans and left a large variety of kids orphaned. Not totally finished, a greater quantity of Americans died of Spanish influenza as compared to World War I; extra died than in all the wars of the 20 th century combined. Universally, the pandemic infected 33% of the planet's population and killed an anticipated 50 million people.

However, for all of the lives out of location and changed all of the time, Spanish influenza rapid faded from public reputation. "It fell into this darkish hollow of records," Davis says. "Affected families in no way appeared to talk masses about it, possibly as it changed into horrible to such an quantity that no one had to reconsider it. That is the way the u . S . Also handled it."

This season's flu virus appeared to hit with a problem of randomness, and cruelly so. Since grown-u.S. Of americainside the excessive of lifestyles died in droves, unfortunate communities collapsed. Kids had been orphaned, older guardians left to fight for themselves. Individuals had been at a loss to make smooth this easy lottery, and it left them deeply disturbed. Attempting to painting the feeling it propelled in him, a French expert in the town of Lyons wrote that it become very awesome to the "intestine pangs" he had skilled on the equal time as serving on the the the front. This changed into "more diffuse tension, the vibe of a few indefinable horror which had taken maintain of the population of that town."

It end up definitely later at the same time as sickness transmission professionals targeted at the numbers that examples began out out to rise, and the principle components of clarification had been superior. A part of the variety is probably clarified by way of way of disparities of wealth and caste, and to the diploma that it contemplated those elements, further to pores and pores and skin color. Bad weight loss program, crowded living, and restricted get proper of access to to human offerings debilitated the constitution, rendering terrible humans, settlers, and ethnic minorities extra liable to disease. As a French scholar of information, Patrick Zylberman placed it: "The infection can also furthermore well have carried on 'democratically,' but the general public it attacked changed into not egalitarian."

Some different underlying ailments made a person more vulnerable to Spanish influenza, while earlier presentation to this season's flu virus itself regulated the severity of a case. Remote people corporation without masses of verifiable experience of the sickness suffered badly, as did city groups that have been bypassed through the usage of the primary wave of the pandemic because of the fact they had been not immunologically 'prepared' for the second one. For example, Rio de Janeiro, the capital of Brazil at that component, have been given certainly one influx of influenza, in October 1918, and experienced a lack of lifestyles price some instances higher than that recorded in American town areas toward the north that had gotten every the spring and autumn waves. And Bristol Bay in Alaska changed into saved till mid-1919, but even as the infection at lengthy very last expanded, it reduced the bay's Eskimo populace via forty%.

Public fitness campaigns didn't have any type of impact, regardless of the truth that surgeons did not understand the purpose for the ailment. Since days of yore, at some factor point sickness is a threat, human beings have polished 'social distancing,' understanding truely that retaining off inflamed people builds the opportunity of last sound. In 1918, social setting aside appeared as isolate regions, isolation wards, and prohibitions on mass get-togethers; wherein they were as it should be upheld, those measures eased again the spread. Australia stored out the harvest time wave altogether by way of the usage of enforcing an powerful quarantine at its ports.

Similarly reliable, but in emotional and intellectual phrases, grow to be the grief introduced approximately via the sudden mass dying which originated from the pandemic. Families broken by means of manner of the use of the death of a young parent or accomplice and orphans, delivered to the damage spilling out of these deaths, lots of the time for the the rest in their lives. In 1998 a ninety-year-vintage South African influenza vagrant observed out to me that his mom had surpassed away inside the 1918 pandemic at the same time as he changed into ten, "and I in reality have unnoticed her from that factor onward. "At the same time a subsequent nonagenarian reviewed powerfully that once his mother had died on of "Spanish" influenza in Illinois in 1918, the sparkle left everything. I understood, sincerely because of the truth and all of the time, that we have been not stable. We had been now not beyond damage. My dad did what he may additionally need to. He saved us all collectively, however from that time on, there has been a pity which had not existed previously, a in which it counts misery that never went away.

In any case, in 1919, most flu widows who had out of place their enterprise enterprise husbands had a quick duration to harp on their loss, being compelled to find out instantaneous methods to assist their kids. Going to their families for assist, stepping into a good deal less high-priced consolation, or entering into the venture market much more likely than not, had now not been an normal enjoy globally for girls in this situation. "My costly companion passed directly to the great past of influenza, leaving me with five youngsters in poverty and debt," conceded one such influenza widow in rustic South Africa. "Petition God for me for recognition and electricity. I intend to visit the diamond diggings to test whether or not or not I can get with the resource of. Approach the Lord for consolation and help. "Many a small scale statistics will be required earlier than historians can exactly guide such patterns and their variations throughout the area.

www.ingramcontent.com/pod-product-compliance
Lightning Source LLC
Chambersburg PA
CBHW071447080526
44587CB00014B/2018
* 9 7 8 1 7 7 5 3 1 4 2 6 4 *